ll
the
best for
the future

All the best for the future

Greg James

Growing Up Without Growing Old

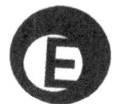

EBURY
SPOTLIGHT

EBURY SPOTLIGHT

UK | USA | Canada | Ireland | Australia
India | New Zealand | South Africa

Ebury Spotlight is part of the Penguin Random House group of companies
whose addresses can be found at global.penguinrandomhouse.com

Penguin Random House UK
One Embassy Gardens, 8 Viaduct Gardens, London SW11 7BW

penguin.co.uk
global.penguinrandomhouse.com

Penguin
Random House
UK

First published by Ebury Spotlight in 2025

1

Typeset by seagulls.net

Printed and bound in Great Britain by Clays Ltd, Elcograf S.p.A.

The authorised representative in the EEA is Penguin Random House Ireland,
Morrison Chambers, 32 Nassau Street, Dublin D02 YH68

A CIP catalogue record for this book is available from the British Library

Hardback ISBN 9781529912197
Trade paperback ISBN 9781529980226

MIX
Paper | Supporting
responsible forestry
FSC
www.fsc.org   FSC® C018179

Penguin Random House is committed to a sustainable future
for our business, our readers and our planet. This book is made
from Forest Stewardship Council® certified paper.

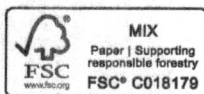

For Alan, Rosemary, Catherine,
Bella and Barney

Contents

From Me, to You

I was getting closer. I was about to meet them. My heroes. Up until this moment, they'd only existed on the TV after a long and arduous day at primary school, but there they were. Actually real. I could hear them in the distance laughing and doing their catchphrases. They sounded like they were on form: they were full of energy, full of laughter. I could see their brightly coloured tops in the distance. As an act of reverence, I too was wearing my brightest shell suit for them. This only came out on special occasions. My god I loved a polyester tracksuit. The more man-made the better. Wipe-clean, comfortable … flammable. In fact, everyone had dressed up for the two titans of nonsense. A sea of bright primary colours as hundreds of children patiently waited, dressed in an array of baggy jumpers, new trainers and loose-fitting trackies. Kappa to the left of me, Fila to the right, here I was, stuck in the middle with them. The room was abuzz. Small pockets of screams and yelps erupted sporadically. It smelt of nervous energy. Farts and crisps, basically. If I could just get to the end of this interminable line, I'd get to meet the oracles in the flesh. I was ten years old so I didn't know what interminable meant. I also didn't know that the next 15 minutes would alter the course of my life. Forever.

Our story opens in Weymouth, in 1996, which by this time was a faded-glory seaside town in Dorset. During the Victorian era, Weymouth was the South of France, Mallorca and Tuscany all rolled into one. It was the place to be. In the summer months at least. The royal family used to holiday there. There's even a clock tower on the seafront to commemorate Queen Victoria's 50 years on the throne. As well as telling the time, its main function nowadays is less a celebration of royal visitors and more a prominent pillar for local dogs to cock a leg up. Not sure Big Vic would be looking down and particularly enjoying that her Golden Jubilee clock gets half-hourly golden showers from the local hounds, but that's life. Or death, in her case. And as the old saying goes: 'You can't stop a dog pissing up your clock tower.' The royals definitely don't go there anymore, though. I mean, one of the shit ones might if they need to catch the ferry to Guernsey to stand around at a regatta or something, but Wills and Kate definitely aren't sploshing around on the bumper boats at Lodmoor or popping in to say hi to the Humboldt penguins at the Sea Life Centre. My mum's side of the family are the reason we went to Weymouth every holiday when I was younger. And I loved it. I'd get to hang out with my three cousins, William, Piran and Guy, who were (and still are) a similar age to me, and my nan and grandad, who were a lot older than me (and are now dead). And they all lived *by the sea*. I was so jealous. What a great life. Well, in June, July and August at least. It's bleak as tits in the winter.

Back to the queue. I'm with my (now dead) nan, waiting nervously but patiently to get an autograph from my comedy heroes after watching – what I thought to be at the time – the greatest show on earth – *The Chuckle Brothers LIVE*. I loved the Chuckle Brothers. I still do. They were silly for the sake of silly. This was early exposure to slapstick, to catchphrases, to anarchy, to nonsense and to that really great pedal car thing they used to bowl around in, spilling tins of paint and knocking over ladders. They were clowns. And brilliant ones at that. They are to me what the Sex Pistols or The Clash are to people who think they're cooler than everyone else. To me, they were punk. The kid in front of me finally cleared off and it was my turn. I shuffled sheepishly towards the signing desk, pen and programme in hand. I panicked that the magnitude of the moment was going to get to me. I was so nervous. But the nerves dissipated as soon as I was greeted by the two brightest and biggest smiles I'd ever seen. 'El-ohhha!' they said in unison. Paul and Barry had developed a unique way of saying 'hello'. With their distinctive Lancashire Yorkshire accents, they managed a little trill on the end that was sort of an 'ah' but is very hard to replicate on the page. If you're lucky enough to have purchased the audiobook of this and you're listening to me read to you, I can tell you exactly what it sounds like. If you're stuck in the dark ages and you're reading these words yourself, the best thing I can suggest is to watch them saying it on YouTube. 'Hello!' I replied excitedly. I immediately clammed up. I panicked. Of course I did. The magnitude of the moment *did* get to me. And that's how it should be. I'm always a little freaked out by those kids that are *too* confident, you know? Why are you already talking like a grown-up? It's a red flag. They're probably using the word 'interminable' to describe the long queue. I can't remember the details of the chat but I imagine I told them my name and said they were really funny and I loved the show. They then grabbed a glossy photo card from the pile next to them and asked me my name. I said, 'Gregory.' I was rocking Gregory back then. Paul started to write:

To Gregory,
All the best for the future,
Love,
Paul and Barry.

I muttered a thank you, and he handed it to me. 'To you,' said Paul. 'To me,' I replied. They chuckled. Of course they did.

My nan thanked them and ushered me away from the grinning brothers. I was stunned. I was ecstatic. As we walked out of the bar area where they were stationed, down the stairs and out into the bright Dorset sunshine, it dawned on me that this was the greatest moment of my life. I'd done one of their catchphrases *with* them. For a brief moment, I was the third, much younger, Chuckle. It was my first face-to-face encounter with showbusiness. And it felt good. Little did that ten-year-old know that one day he'd also be making parents and grandparents wait for fucking ages in order for their kids to nervously come up to a rickety signing table, receive a signed book and exchange a silly catchphrase of his own. 'Are you well? I thought you were.' 'Oh, and give my regards to your lizard.'

That ten-year-old didn't really know anything. How could he? He had no idea how life would pan out. We started the walk back to Nan's along the seafront, or 'The Esplanade', as the locals insist on calling it, past the clock tower as another dog was in full flow and my nan asked to have a look at the autograph. 'To Gregory, All the best for the future,' she read out loud. 'That's a weird thing to say to a ten-year-old, isn't it?!'

I didn't think that at the time. I didn't really think anything at the time apart from I'd had a nice afternoon watching some funny men splatting each other with custard pies for a couple of hours. I was also thinking about whether Nan would let me get McDonald's on the way back to hers. But on reflection, I agree with her. 'All the best for the future' is a fucking mad thing to say to a child. But it's also hilarious. It's oddly formal. The sort of thing you'd say in the leaving card of a colleague you barely know. But from them, to little me, it's funny. It's a grand statement to a small boy which means simultaneously everything and also nothing. And I still remember it vividly and it makes me laugh every time I think about it. Ten-year-old Gregory had no idea what was in store for him as his life panned out. No one knows what's coming. And that's really the point of this book. You might have had (and you still might have) huge plans. Specific plans. Big dreams. Little dreams. Ideas about how your life might end up. Fantasies about how it will go. When you'll get married, where you'll live, how many children you want, what job you'll end up doing. But really, we're not in control of much of it. And as a concept that can be hard and upsetting to deal with. But life can also be beautifully surprising and take a course you never imagined. I want this book to serve as a companion for you if you ever need a reminder of this. And hopefully something to make you laugh and remind you to try your best to always find the fun.

Over the next few hundred pages, I'll cover the big life things, the things that wind me up, the things that make me sad, the things that make me laugh and the little things, passions and interests that we all rely on to get us through the day – whether it was a good one or a bad one. I also want to tell you a bit about who I actually am, who I thought I'd be and who I think I still could be. You might have listened to me on the radio for years but even then, you've only really been exposed to a small percentage of me. People are many things. For example, I can be incredibly grumpy, I scream when someone wakes me up from any sleep, when I'm sad or anxious I'll watch a James Bond film, I am prone to huge bouts of self-doubt, I love very sad music, I crave physical contact and I am a tragic nostalgist. We're all guilty of reducing each other to simple caricatures and one of my aims is to let you in on a few other bits of my life in the hope it'll give you confidence to express yourself fully and not be inhibited by what the world or your family or your friends want you to be like. I started writing this book as a reminder to myself to always continue to seek out the fun and to never lose sight of or move away from my true passions and interests.

Without wanting to cause you to spiral into an existential crisis, I found that realising there isn't an ultimate and final destination in life made living it a lot easier. I mean, there is an ultimate end point, I guess. Eventually we'll all end up as ashes thrown off your favourite cliff. Or memorialised with a commemorative bench overlooking your favourite cliff. Or laid to rest in a cemetery next to a man called Cliff. You get the idea. But don't dwell on that too much. Oh, hang on, I've managed to spin that positive thought into a bleak one. Let's do as Pitbull would do and turn that negative into a positive. Dale!

Mantras tend to be clichéd and oversimplistic, I realise that. Before you know it you've bought a 'Live, Laugh, Love' cushion and you're singing about 'living each day as if it's your last' and telling everyone that 'it takes more muscles to frown than it does to smile'. But if I was to try to come up with a mantra, it would be something like, 'Try to do some fun shit before you run out of time if you possibly can.' But that's not particularly catchy and your aunty would hate it if you bought her cushion covers with that plastered across.

Obviously most of us need to work to be able to afford life and a decent job makes it easier, but getting the balance of work and play right is something we all struggle with. Becoming an adult, for the most part, is really fucking hard work and it's a complete shock to the system when it's suddenly all on *you*. Not only do you have to hold down a job where you give the illusion of being a fully functioning, fully formed human being at all times but you also might have to juggle kids, a partner, mortgages, rent, council tax, the food shop, booking things, cancelling things, re-booking things, fixing the roof, cutting the grass, washing up, hoovering, taking the dog for a walk … you get the idea. All the while, when is there time or space for you to prioritise some of the things that you're truly passionate about? The things that make you, you. Just because you're getting older, it doesn't mean you have to get *old* and forget about all the things you loved doing before you became an adult.

It's all too easy for work to become our whole world. We are not defined by what we do as a job. Lots of things make up a life and I'm partly writing this book as a reminder to myself to keep the balance in check. I'm guilty of working too much. I've turned a lot of my hobbies into jobs. I loved listening to the radio so decided to be on it. I adore cricket with my whole being so I started the *Tailenders* podcast and now I get to talk about it once a week with other cricket tragics. I liked reading books so much that I started writing stories for kids. And as wonderfully fortunate as that is, I have to watch that I don't overdo it and end up with no time off to pursue *other* interests and end up with no real personality. And zero friends.

I want to take you through some of my observations of the world and give you my thoughts on some of the big life cross-roads and choices we're all confronted with along the way – and hopefully encourage you to take a look back at what you were like as a kid. What excited you? What were you obsessed with? We shouldn't lose touch with our younger selves because that person will probably be a good reminder to prioritise the things that have always made you truly happy.

This isn't one of those books that will encourage you to blow your life up, by the way. But I do think that along with forgetting about our childhood passions and interests, we're all so busy that sometimes we sleepwalk into quite big commitments without truly working out if it's what we want to be doing. There's a temptation to do things because you *should* instead of doing them because you *want to*. Just to say, there are no right or wrong answers. You could well be very happy living the life you always thought you'd have, but that definitely won't be the case for everyone. We're all in a massive rush to grow up and reach the key milestones of life. School – job – marriage – bigger job – house – bigger house – baby – even bigger job – bigger baby – even bigger house – retire – no job – all your babies leave you – smaller house – dead – won't work for everyone. And nor should it. It's less scary to think that life is like *Mario Kart*, with things to collect, banana skins to avoid checkpoints to zoom through, levels to unlock. And, at times, it can be like that. But crucially, I think it's best not to approach life as if it's a race. Because it isn't. And it's a shame that we're partly conditioned to hurry through life's checkpoints; some of us pushed through them without even giving it a second thought, let alone a critical one.

The notion of 'growing up' itself is probably quite unhelpful. Growing is largely seen as a good thing. I suppose it is. Trees growing big and strong is nice. Same with people. But I know loads of happy short people. I've also seen loads of happy tiny trees. Conversely, 'growing' is bad if it's Japanese knotweed. Or verrucas. So let's not just assume that 'growing' is always good. Or necessary. Or simple.

What's the rush then?! Why are we so desperate to get older? It seems that every kid in my life is hellbent on making sure they're ageing as quickly as possible. How many times have you been furiously corrected when you've had to guess a kid's age and you don't supply the months too?! 'I'm six and seven months, *actually*, Uncle Greg!' Oh pipe down, you precocious turd. Adults should start doing it just to creep people out. Why do we often fall into the trap of wishing away our younger years by racing into adulthood, getting our ears pierced and driving cars, but at the same time also think we have to become more serious?

'Oh, grow up!' we're told if we're being childish and fun. Right, so when we do grow up, fun isn't allowed? I love the idea of getting less and less serious the more you age. I'm actively trying to do that, but it's not easy and you don't just stumble into that frame of mind. You obviously have to give consideration to some of the serious life things I mentioned above, but once you've done that and have made peace with what you can control, the rest of the time could be set aside for play. And that's where I can help. Hopefully.

As I traverse the adult world, it's really easy to become detached from that excited, joyful, naive kid who was waiting impatiently for the Chuckle Brothers. But that is still me. That really is the essence of me. That's maybe the most me I've ever been. It's easy to get so bogged down in adult life that you forget to have fun. I reckon we're all guilty of forgetting to 'prioritise pleasure', as the brilliant Self Esteem says. I'm here to help you unlock those things that make you *you*, in case you've drifted a bit. Because I bet there's something you loved when you were ten that would still make you happy if you revisited it. As I approached my late twenties and early thirties, I consciously leant into the things that made me *me* all those years ago when I was falling in love with comedy, music, sport and nerdy hobbies. And it turns out you can be a fully functioning adult with bills to pay and kids or dogs to look after and still find time to play with a train set. As one of my favourite artists, Mr Bingo, says, don't forget to have fun. I want to encourage you to take fun seriously.

So, thank you for picking up this book. I've really poured my heart and soul into it over the last couple of years. Reading it may completely change your life. And in that case, it's 20 quid well spent. Or £11.99 if you bought it from Amazon because they run the world and are able to undercut everyone, meaning no one makes any money from it apart from them. Thanks a lot, Jeff Bezos. And well done again on that space mission; everyone thought it was brilliant and in no way depressingly dystopian and a complete waste of money. There's a chance that this book doesn't change your life and I'm prepared for that, but what I do hope happens by reading this is that you ask yourself some of the questions I'm going to put to you and, in turn, you might learn a bit more about what you like, what you want to do in your life or, more importantly, what you *don't* want to do. I want to make sure you're still finding time to play, time to embrace the things that gave you joy when you were younger and started you on the path to the person that's reading these words right now. This is as guru-y as I'm going to get, by the way. But more than that, as I do on the radio, I will be trying my very best to make you laugh and have a nice time. I want you to get to the end of this book and have an even better idea of who you are. And in the spirit of that, let me try to answer that question myself. Who the fuck am I?!

The Murder of Greg Milward

Wikipedia thinks it's got me nailed but it doesn't know the full story. Firstly, I'm not Greg James. Well, I am. I've been Greg James for longer than I haven't but it was a name I started using on student radio in 2004. My full name is Gregory James Alan Milward. Yes, that much is on Wikipedia but it's actually a relief to write that down. It's often felt like a dirty secret but actually the origin story makes me laugh whenever someone asks me about it, so I don't know why I haven't ever properly addressed it. It's appeared in the odd interview or profile piece but I've largely just ignored it/him and perhaps I was embarrassed by it/him but now, over 20 years later, I've had all shame beaten out of me by showbusiness.

It was the autumn of 2004, the setting: the University of East Anglia. Freshers' fair. And a beanstalk of a man called Dave Bradshaw lumbered up to me outside the Brutalist concrete block that was the student union and asked if I wanted to join Livewire 1350 AM (UEA's home of new music), the student radio station on campus. Of course I did. Yes, the fact that I could do English and Drama two hours away from home, which was far enough away to feel like I was being adventurous but not too far in case I couldn't find any friends or needed my washing done, was very attractive. But so was the presence of a student radio station. Obviously I'd checked on that before submitting my UCAS form. I knew I'd find it at some point. I just didn't expect to do so in hour one of day one. This encounter with Big Dave inadvertently changed the course of my entire life and simultaneously killed off its main character – him, Greg Milward, RIP. Dave Bradshaw was the murderer. More on that later.

I immediately went upstairs to meet the third years, who were having the time of their lives in the fully decked-out *live* radio studios. This was it. This was the place that immediately felt like home. I get quite emotional thinking about it. I remember it so vividly.

Livewire was situated on the top floor of Union House over-looking the campus and consisted of two studios that were littered with CDs without cases, tangled wires, old wheezing computers and, most excitingly, fully functioning and surprisingly professional radio desks. It was heaven. Faders, buttons, dials, knobs, micro-phones, CD players, a computer for playing clips and jingles. I couldn't believe it. Strewn across the walls were posters of bands that had recently played downstairs at The LCR and in among them were signatures of celebrities and artists that had been interviewed on the radio station. The Libertines, Kings of Leon and The Yeah Yeah Yeahs are some I remember from that first visit. It was scuzzy, unrefined, full of old equipment, racks of dusty copies of *NME*, stacks of vinyl and cupboards full of promotional tat. It was busy, vibrant, smelled of chips and teenagers and it was the most magical place I'd ever set foot in. Radio at its most pure and unfussy.

Along with Dave, I met Francis Hamlyn and Simon Williams, who immediately became my best radio friends. Oooh radio friends. We spent the next few years making shows together, putting on club nights, interviewing new bands, setting up outside broadcasts and generally arsing around and learning the basics of how to run a radio station.

It was a complete joy from start to finish. Some of the happiest memories of my life. I'd found the radio nerds. To my mind, they were the coolest people on campus. But, of course, they were anything but cool. They were absolute eggheads, all of them. Big virgin energy. It was fantastic. They made ME feel cool. I'd hit the jackpot and found my tribe.

I was no longer embarrassed to say I loved radio and that I wanted to do it as a job one day. I used to be ashamed of everything I loved when I was a teenager. I loved acting. I really wanted to be an actor. I still sort of do, actually. I also loved singing. But even now I feel hesitant to admit that I was in the school choir when I was a kid. I loved being in the choir but was mortified if anyone spotted me in the music room. Kids are insane. We're all insane. Why are we like this? What the fuck were we worried about? Was I careful who I told about those passions? Did I hide them from people? You're damn right I did. Why? Aside from the fear of getting bullied by repressed thick twats, I have no idea. Singing and acting are two of the coolest jobs. Actors and musicians are among the most revered and respected people on earth. We all love actors. We all love singers. For example, at the time of writing, the world can be split into those who want to have sex with Jonathan Bailey and those that want to be best friends with Taylor Swift. Why is it that we're OK telling everyone we love these people but are terrified of anyone finding out we might want to *be* them?

But back to the murder of Greg Milward ... In order to get a slot in the Livewire schedule for the upcoming term, you had to write a show brief, with some sample ideas and explaining the style of music you'd play, and submit a short demo tape of you in the studio pretending to do a show. Obviously, I made sure I absolutely smashed this brief with a mixture of features robbed from Scott Mills, delivered in the style of Ricky Gervais and accompanied by the playlist from XFM in its indie heyday, all the while taking notes from watching the first series of *I'm Alan Partridge*, in which Alan is on Radio Norwich. In fact, *I'm Alan Partridge* was my favourite show not only because it was the funniest thing I'd ever seen but also because it was my first look inside a radio station. Armando Iannucci, one of the creators of Partridge and a comedy hero of mine, actually started his career on the radio at BBC Scotland. As soon as I saw the level of detail in Alan's fake studio, I knew it could have only been created by a proper radio nerd. The desk, the clocks, the faders and mics were all, as we say in the industry ... 'industry standard'.

On the application form for Livewire, I vividly remember writing my name out: GREG JAMES. It was a bit of a joke really. I fancied a DJ name. Milward isn't a DJ name. It's just not. It's a good name for a headteacher. Just ask my dad, the retired headteacher Alan Milward. But it's not very Radio 1, is it? SCOTT MILLS. Good radio name. ZANE LOWE (real name Alexander Zane Lowe). GREAT name. SARA COX. Again, amazing. GREG MILWARD. No. Sorry, next. So, I killed him. Quickly and painlessly. In hindsight, I could have been a bit more adventurous. In creating my new identity I only ventured as far as my middle name, which doesn't scream 'creative powerhouse', does it? What would have been more exciting? GREG MAGIC. GREG VOLCANO. GREG BLAST. GREG STORM. Could have gone quirky: GREG GREGSON, GREG GREGORY, GREG TALL, COUSIN GREG, GREG WOW, GREGORIAN CALENDAR, GREGGINGTON WORLD OF ADVENTURES. All good options and yet I chose GREG JAMES. I really love having an alter ego. I've been called that since I was 18. The only people that 'Greg Milward' me are the bank, EDF Energy (who I hate) and the police (who very rarely contact me). GREG JAMES accidentally became a permanent fixture in my life when I won a Student Radio Award and part of the prize was to do a one-hour show on Radio 1 in 2005. I won the award as Greg James. And before I could really even think about it, that name appeared in the *Radio Times* and that was it. I was on air to millions of people as him. Or rather, me. I've been him, or he's been me, ever since. Is there any difference? Maybe at first it gave me confidence to play a role. Looked at another way, I've been in deep cover as a radio presenter called Greg James for 20 years. It's been the role of a lifetime. Hopefully I've been convincing. But who's who? And who are these people? Maybe we should try to unpack that. Probably a useful task. But perhaps a daunting one. To quote my mum when I urged her to go and have therapy – 'oh no, I don't fancy that. What if they dig up something uncomfortable?!'

I was born on 17 December 1985 at Lewisham Hospital in south London. Yes, I'm old, 39 at the time of typing. Please alter the age depending on when you're reading this. For example, if you're reading this before 17 December 2025, I'm 39. Anytime up until 17 December 2026, I'll be 40. And so on. If I've tragically died and you bought this because I'm being celebrated on a series of special broadcasts across the BBC and you've only just realised how brilliant I am, then I am still the age I was when I died. That happens to lots of people, doesn't it. It might happen to me. People only truly realised how lucky we were to have Bowie when he wasn't around anymore. A similar thing happened when they threatened to kill BBC Radio 6 Music. No one really gave it a second thought until they threatened to close it and everyone complained and it was saved. Thank fuck. I've got distracted but I guess what I'm saying is in terms of cultural significance, I sit somewhere between David Bowie and 6 Music.

But before I was Greg James and knew who David Bowie even was, I was just a kid. A normal kid. Kid Normal, if you will. It's weird being a child. If an adult friend behaved like a two-year-old, you'd intervene, wouldn't you? When my wife, Bella, and I were on holiday recently with Bella's sister and her two-year-old son, he ate a peach, two tomatoes and a slice of shepherd's pie for lunch and then went to bed for four hours. That's unhinged. He hadn't got a fucking clue what was going on. It's a nice life, though, isn't it. My nephew has all of us fawning over him, peaches on tap, talking to him like he's a very clever deaf dog. Applauding when he smiles and finishes a drink without tipping it over his head, or mine. You're a mess when you're two. Or maybe we're a mess at every age.

The thing that always baffles me with kids that age is that they'll never remember any of it. He'll be able to piece it all together with the extensive collection of photos and videos we've all taken of him but you don't remember what it's like to be two. The people that tell you they remember what it's like are lying, by the way. There's no way to critically analyse your early years. What sort of kid were you? Did you have a nice time? Were you annoying? He's a good one, though, a really good one. Laith, one day you'll realise this bit of the book is about you and you'll also realise how much of a national treasure your uncle is/was. Anyway, he's a very sweet child and objectively not a rubbish one. It's awful when your friends or family have a shit kid. It's such a shame, isn't it? No one talks about it – but everyone knows deep down that you've got a bad one. A screamy one. A miserable one. A dictator. One that disrupts every adult interaction by throwing a glass on the floor or having a meltdown because the iPad was taken away. But whether you were a baby Hitler or a … baby … Teresa (Mother, not May), you won't remember any of it at all.

Children are always desperate to grow up, to be a big boy or girl. When does it change from this to 'Holy hell I hate this, why am I so incredibly elderly and decrepit? Oh shit, I'm going to die soon?' I think there are stages. And I think you regress and progress as you go through them. This stuff isn't straightforward. But from one to four, you're essentially a waste of space. If you're lucky, a cute waste of space, but a waste of space all the same. You're not adding much to the world on any scale. Four to ten I'd say is prime 'I want to be older' territory. You're talking, you're starting to find things funny, you're doing impressions of your parents, you've got a favourite Disney film, you start getting good at sport, you're reading. And by 'reading' I of course mean that you use your parent's phone to go on TikTok and start that long and toxic relationship with social media. But, despite that, you think you're pretty fly by ten.

Ten to thirteen is tricky, isn't it? I remember hating the idea of being a teenager. The specific reasons for this will be discussed in a later chapter that will confirm to you what a fucking loser I was. But I think I quite liked being eleven, specifically. Eleven was a good year for me. I was good at computer stuff, I loved messing around making little films on a camcorder, I was really good at cricket, I enjoyed hanging out with my parents, I started properly falling in love with radio and pop music, I started riding a bike everywhere, I had a great remote-controlled car, nice friends … life was good. Then thirteen came around. Then fourteen. Oh, sweet Jesus. A horrible mess of wanting to still be that fresh-faced, sweet, happy-go-lucky eleven-year-old but now with weird hair growing everywhere. Honestly, what an insane process. You wait and wait for signs that you're maturing and growing up, hoping it might be an instant, striking signal to the world that you're becoming a man, and all you get are pubes. Oh, and your voice completely changes. And you get spots. You start getting really grouchy and you start to smell. Thanks a lot, God. In fact this is just another reason why I've never once believed in him/her. I added 'her' because I know a lot of the people who like me are women. I am an ally. Remember that. Even for your stupid fucking lady god that doesn't exist.

By 15, I just wanted it all to stop. I couldn't bear it. I would have been so happy to jump from 11 straight to 17. The years between were awful. And it wasn't because I desperately wanted to be old, it was because I just desperately wanted to be sorted. I didn't enjoy being a teenager that much. I guess this is pretty common but it didn't feel like it at the time. I felt like others wore being a teenager really lightly whereas I was wearing a heavy, uncomfortable cloak of awkwardness over a body I had to shuffle around in for a few years.

I didn't fit in as a teenager but maybe that's just teenagers: they don't fit in because they're all monsters bursting out of kids' clothes. To me, everyone else seemed like they had their shit together, though. Some did, some didn't, I guess. Other people my age looked like they were ready to grow up, they were embracing their adolescence. My teens were a load of years where I just didn't really know what to do. I still did most of the things I did when I was 11 or 12. I don't suppose that's too radical. It's only a matter of a few years and I'm still the same person now that I was at 35, for example. But somehow in your teens, a few years is like a lifetime: you morph into an entirely different person altogether. I felt pressured to grow up but I wasn't ready to. And I didn't want to. I liked my life as it was, I was content. At the time, however, I wished I was able to just automatically 'be cool'. It seemed like lots of kids in my year found this very easy. I just couldn't and instead focused on doing things I enjoyed. Of course, in hindsight, I'm so pleased I did. Turns out, I was accidentally doing it right! I liked all the things I was doing and all the hobbies I'd started, and being an adult seemed like hard work. My dad would always be home late and be stressed, my mum was often charging around getting stuff done and there was often talk in the house about debt and overdrafts and mortgages, which sounded worrying but also dull. I was much happier watering the front path when it was below freezing to give my remote-controlled car a skid pan. I still miss those days. Might do that this evening, actually. I got a new R/C car for my birthday from my mate Jonny.

Reappraising that period now, though, I'm pleased I didn't do too much stuff I didn't want to. I played it relatively safe until I worked out what I was all about. I didn't need to make too many big mistakes, fall out with my parents or take a load of drugs. In fact, I really didn't want to move away from Mum and Dad until I got to the end of sixth form. Those two years really were the making of me. I was clearly a late developer but by 17 or 18, I discovered a new confidence. A confidence in not only what I enjoyed and wanted to spend time doing but also a confidence to be who I was. I think if you were to speak to people who knew me at 18, they'd say that I'm still pretty much the same person. Just with better hair and clothes. And a book deal. And a great old car. (E34 BMW M5, for the nerds reading.)

So, let's get back to the timeline. From four to ten, I was keen to get older. From ten to seventeen, I just wanted to stay a kid and now eighteen? Well, I was very keen to remain eighteen actually. Twenty felt like you were a proper adult but eighteen felt fun. In fact, I think about being that age quite often. I've thought about it a lot while writing this book actually. I was really uninhibited and fearless at eighteen. I didn't desperately want to grow up but I was more convinced that I could become an adult on my terms. I gained confidence to embrace all the things I fell in love with as a kid but also started to realise that I could maybe pursue them in an even more meaningful way. Maybe I could just play forever? I started to read up about adults that did fun jobs and went off to university to do a deliberately semi-serious English and drama degree (English is serious, drama isn't) which still had room for potential nonsense. I was obsessed with comedy, radio and essentially any type of performing. I wanted to be a stand-up come-dian, a sit-down radio presenter and a laid-back movie star all at once. I wanted to do everything. And I thought I could do it. That mindset, although exhausting if you're like that all the time, is really crucial for doing the jobs that I do.

I go back to that 'place' as often as I can to remember to enjoy everything and to not get bogged down in the mundanities of adult life. This whole book serves as a reminder to all of us to try to remember the first time you realised you loved something or found a passion. What's that thing you do for fun? When are you most playful and most joyful? Do that! As much as you can! You don't have to make it into a job. I was lucky that these passions and ambi-tions coalesced for me when I was 18 and on my good days, I'm still that boy. I only write bits of this book when I feel like him. I'm a lot smarter and better at writing now than I was at 18 (as I should be), but my approach to life and work, which was so simple and raw back then, is still the same. And it came from a really honest place of *I just want to have a nice time and make some fun things.* That's what I try and hold on to. You can find your own version of this. That version of you before being an adult completely took hold. It's crucial. And also fun. Because being 'an adult' doesn't really *mean* anything. You're you. You've always been that. And you always will be. Oh god, that's *very* self-help, isn't it. Hang on, let me undercut it with a funny line … You will always be you … until you die. And then you'll be nothing and none of this will have mattered.

Life is simultaneously short and long. I think that might be the beauty of it. The summer holidays are the perfect example of this. Six weeks long, unless you went to a posh school. I was going to write 'unless you were a posh twat' but realised that a lot of people who like me are posh twats because I like cricket, so I softened it. And in any case, there are some really nice posh twats knocking around. For most schools, the holidays were six weeks long and at the start of it all, mid-July, it feels like you'll never have to go back. I remember gliding around the corridors as I emptied my locker saying farewell to my teachers and the people in my form who I didn't like with a gleeful 'Goodbye forever!' smile. Maybe if I was lucky I'd get to have a couple of weeks in the sunshine and for the rest of the time I'd go and see Nan, Grandad and my cousins in Weymouth or waste hours watching summer telly (thank you, T4) while eating bowl after bowl of Shreddies, play a bit of cricket, watch the *Big Brother* live stream all day, see a few mates and next thing you know it's getting dark a bit earlier, all the shops have depressing back-to-school displays and you've got to get your head around a new timetable. Before you know it, you're back in your form room sitting next to that prick Tom Faiers again like nothing happened. The holidays are over in a flash. Like life, I guess. But within that are hours upon hours of nothing. No real worries. Nothing much to do. Care-free. I really hate the phrase 'youth is wasted on the young' but honestly, I really did waste those six weeks. But maybe the real winners with school holidays are the teachers. They deserve that break. Can you imagine what you'd do if suddenly your boss said, 'All right, we're doing a summer holiday this year. Six weeks off. See you in September.' The amount of shit you'd get done! I'd panic and immediately think I had to travel the world. I'd learn a new language, write a few more books, get divorced, remarry, divorce again and then grovel to get Bella back. That sort of thing. But actually, that's a very 'grown-up' way of approaching it. Kids, meanwhile, are great at doing a fat load of nothing. Adults tend to have an inbuilt pressure to make the most of the time and be practical. But really, we should learn from our teenage selves. It's vital that we let ourselves get bored, whatever age we are. We've become less good at that the more obsessed with social media we've become. Kids need to be given time off from learning to make sure playing and resting is prioritised. But as adults, why do we set unachievable aims for our time off? The best thing to do in those six weeks would be to relax. Have some dead days. Give yourself some time to rest and get bored, just mess around with something you find enjoyable. On a recent week-long holiday, I took six books with me. SIX! It's absurd. And obviously I didn't read any of them. They looked nice on my bedside table, though. Aesthetically, it was a great idea. But I also looked at them every day. There they were, hundreds of characters trapped between the covers judging me for not bothering to get to know them. But I couldn't be arsed. And that's actually OK, as I was knackered.

We're forced to see life as a series of levels to graduate to. Each passing year is a new one to be completed. School reinforces this by making you move 'up' the school. 'New level UNLOCKED! ... You can now enter Year 9!' OK, now what?! Well, you keep going. You get older and another new level is unlocked and then another. You're allowed to drive at 17. You can drink at 18. Then you can leave school and ... Oh, Christ – you've got maybe 70 more years to play with. We're primed to start searching for more levels to achieve by our earlier experiences of school, exams and achievements. Do more! Keep going! Keep striving! Keep hustling! It's very 'crypto bro', isn't it? It's nice to have ambitions and dreams but I don't know if it's healthy to measure ourselves, our happiness and our success on achieving these milestones on this predetermined path that we all feel we have to tread. Do we stop and question it and consider if it is what we want? Do you actually WANT to do all the things you think you should be doing? 'There's more than one way to skin a cat', as the mad old saying goes. Weird graphic cat analogy aside, the point is that there's more than one way to do life. But don't worry about the bigger picture for now. You're having a great time reading this hilarious and insightful book. I'm going to suggest you take a break right now. Why should kids be the only ones that are allowed to do sweet fuck all with their time? Treat yourself. Let's be slobs together.

The Art of Doing Fuck All

When was the last time you did fuck all and didn't panic or feel bad about it? There's a huge expectation on all of us that we have to constantly be 'on', forever busy, always on the move. So much of the modern world has been designed to command our attention that it's almost impossible to switch off completely or get to a point of not having things to do. But if you find yourself with a free day ahead of you, perhaps every now and then, don't arrange anything. Daunting, isn't it, the idea of staring into the abyss on an unremarkable Sunday? When I was a kid, there would be days where all I'd achieve would be eating Coco Pops and riding my bike up and down the cul-de-sac. The glory days. And I mean that seriously. What a life that was. Well, guess what, grown-ups? You can still do that. Not every day, obviously – your friends will start to worry. But really, what's stopping you removing yourself from the world for the day? And how about this for a revolutionary idea – don't tell anyone you're doing it. Don't even post about it online. Just do a nice quiet thing for *yourself.*

Yeah, I know you might have a dog or a kid or something annoying like that – responsibilities blah blah blah blah. But! Plan! Get rid of the kid or the dog for the afternoon. And piss off to go and do a fat load of nothing. Surprise yourself with how useless you've been. Make yourself laugh with how absurdly dull you can make your day. Make a mockery of the exhausting capitalist nightmare world we've created where you can't leave the house without your phone anymore *because your bank card is on it*. Stick two fingers up at whoever it is that's trapped us here in this fast-lane nightmare life. Here are some ideas of what you could do with your time, inspired by my own dream days.

* Spend a day eating bread. For me, it would be onion bagels, tiger bread or if I'm feeling fancy I'll go for challah: a Jewish sweet, soft bread that goes very well with an entire tub of Lurpak. Just have a loaf on the go all day and pop back for pit stops throughout.

* Watch some films that make you happy. It could be a perfect time to catch up on the several years of buzzy Oscars films you've missed. Or watch the same old films you love again. Personally I'd go for *Life of Brian*, any Pierce Brosnan Bond film or the funniest film of all time, *Airplane!* You haven't asked for a recommendation but while I've got you, my friend Fred recommended a film to me called *Toni Erdmann* and it changed my life. It might just be the most brilliant film I've ever seen. It won't be to everyone's taste as it's quite long and doesn't have car chases or lots of tits (it has a few) but it's a beautiful reminder to make sure you don't take life too seriously as you get older. It resonated with me so much and is essentially the core message of this book, too.

* Get in the bath. Start the day with a breakfast bath while eating the aforementioned bread, or maybe branch out to a croissant. Add coffee. Sit there and listen to an album you

like. Maggie Rogers's music is good for bathing. I don't know whether she'd like that review. The latest album from a brilliant band called Divorce is really good soaking music too. Plus the new Self Esteem one if you want to feel like a powerful woman, like me. Ludovico Einaudi is also a good bet for a bath. Or writing. (I wrote all of this book while listening to his music.) A lunchtime bath or a dinner bath are also good. I've been known to Deliveroo a pad thai to coincide with the bubbles reaching their optimum altitude. Normalise the pad Thai bubble bath please. If you don't have a bath, earnestly ask a friend who does have one if you can use it for the day. Their reaction alone will be worth it. Alternatively, perhaps it's time for a trip home to see your parents. No doubt they'll be boomers and they'll have a bath because they got lucky with the housing market in the 1980s.

★ Read a book. Take all day doing it and indulge in it taking ages and it being hard. Don't fret if you don't finish it. No one cares. You can pick something you know you'll enjoy or pick something new and if you hate it, don't see it as a failure. It's so mad to me that we will happily start watching a film and if it's shit, turn it off and get on with your life, guilt free, but if we read a book and think the same, we'll keep going. There isn't any shame in hating a book. Except this one. If you hate this one, you're wrong and stupid and you should be ashamed. Because you're a failure. You must keep going and never tell anyone you don't like it because they'll just laugh at you. In fact they won't believe you anyway so just shut up and keep reading, OK?

* Catch a train, jump on a bus or get in the car and go somewhere new. Even if it's only a couple of stops or a few miles away. When you get there, wander around a bit, go and have a solo drink and a packet of Bacon or Scampi Fries in the oldest pub you can find, sit in silence without your phone or talk to the landlady or landlord or a mad-looking local and then go home. Life doesn't always have to be profound or amazing or meaningful. Every now and then it can and should be dull and unremarkable. Revel in that.

* Spend the day writing some stuff down. Then burn it at all. Honestly, just write the words that form in your head. A thought you have about work or your friend or the person you're in love with. The burning bit is dramatic, but funny. You'll think you're in an episode of *Luther* or something. But dear god don't let anyone see what you've written. Be prepared to immediately leave the country if it falls into the wrong hands. Mortifying.

There you go. Some ideas to get you started and now it is over to you: I can't spoon-feed you everything. But we do need to come up with a name for one of these days. Goblin Mode is one that makes me laugh whenever I see it mentioned. Rotting is also funny. A Waste Day is also quite nice.

You know what. I'm going to have a Waste Day and write the exact timetable for you here. Really, I should be working. But also, I'm only writing a stupid book so it's hardly a real job. Enjoy! I can finally fulfill my dream of doing one of those wellness books where all you do is write a heading and make the reader do the rest. Nice work if you can get it, eh? I've always wanted to write one of those books and have a few pages set aside for really stupid things, like:

'Hey guys! In this chapter, I want you to focus on the five people you hate most in the world and why. Off you go!'

Something like that. Not a bad idea actually. I'm going to call my editor and ask if I can put one in this book. Hang on.

. . .

. . .

. . .

She's not into it.

'Well, it's your book and I can't stop you from writing what you want, but I do think it would be best to keep it positive and uplifting,' she said.

The Five People I Hate the Most in the World

1. Charlotte Hardman (my editor)
2.
3.
4.
5.

Anyway. Here is my Completely Pointless Day of Nothing Much. I've chosen a day when I'm on my summer holidays in the South of France. This feels like an extra fancy version of a waste day but I am quite fancy. It doesn't have to be when you are away but I just wanted to make sure I was properly relaxing and that tends to be when I'm not in radio mode and instead living the life of an elderly Frenchman. This all played out yesterday. Thursday, 13 June 2024:

8.23am – An unplanned early get-up. They're resurfacing the road outside the place we're staying in. The sleepiest village you could imagine but there's a comical dispute ongoing between the water company and the local council about the state of the tarmac. They laid a new surface three days ago then the water lads came and dug up a pipe because there was a problem. This pattern has been happening for six days now. And every morning they're either laying a new road or digging it up again. I don't know if it'll ever get done. Either way, it's fucking noisy. So I'm up.

8.45am – I decided to continue my real-life exercise routine even on holiday. This consists of a 30-minute floor-based routine with a couple of dumbbells. Three, if you include me. I have to do anything I can to distract myself from the act of working out because it's so interminably boring. But completely necessary. I don't want to be old and immobile. To distract myself, I put on an episode of the greatest television show of all time – Michael Palin's *Around the World in 80 Days*. There's a copy of it on DVD in the place we're staying. I couldn't believe my luck. If you've been following me for a while, you'll know I'm completely obsessed with this man. Maybe he deserves a chapter. A chapter on heroes isn't a bad idea. Yeah, I'll come back to him later.

9.45am – Finish my workout as Michael pulls up to Venice and helps out a couple of local refuse collectors. What a lovely man.

10.15am – Yoghurt with berries followed by eggs and French bread soldiers. *Vive la Résistance!* Head back to watch another episode of *Around the World in 80 Days*.

Noon (*midi*) – Still watching *Around the World in 80 Days*. Michael's now in Egypt. I'm still on the sofa eating bread.

1pm – Eating flan. Let's talk about flan, shall we? I've travelled a bit and to my knowledge, the only place that does flan specifically like the stuff I'm obsessed with is … France. It's pretty much the main reason why this is my favourite country. If I could live here, I would. There's often confusion when I talk about flan because lots of people immediately envisage a sort of crème caramel type of character. This is *not* what I mean. Nor do I mean a custard tart. It's not quite that. You're getting close though. It's almost impossible to find in the UK. Believe me, I've tried *very* hard. What I'm talking about is the stuff you can get very cheaply in an Intermarché or E. Leclerc. It's bog-standard, mass-produced, full of sugar, eggy, wobbly flan. It has a very thin, soft, *non*-flaky pastry casing and is served in triangle slices. And my god it's perhaps the most delicious thing anyone's ever made. So yeah, I'm eating that.

2pm – Still here. Michael's just gone through the very narrow Suez Canal. Another slice of floppy flan has gone into my face, thus making my arteries as thin as the canal I'm watching on DVD.

2.30pm – Finally shower.

2.45pm – Fully dry in a matter of minutes because it's 26°C today. Sorry, this country is just better than ours. Yeah, sure, there's a surge in far-right lunatic parties gaining political ground across the country but the weather and the abundance of flan just about redress the balance.

3pm – Have a little snooze. Everyone's aunty on holiday always calls them siestas, don't they? No matter what country you're in.

Also, a big fan of closing for lunch for TWO HOURS. This still happens in rural parts of France. Amazing.

4pm – Pack up the car and head to the beach. The best time to be on the beach is 4pm onwards. Can't be doing with midday madness. Also, I don't want skin cancer, thanks.

4.30pm – Make a deal with the nice man that you hire sunbeds from. He says we can have one of them free because we're there late in the day. It's still €20 though. I decide not to argue because he looks quite hard and my French isn't good enough if I get into an argument.

5.30pm – Get stuck into a book that my good friend and long-time children's book collaborator Chris Smith got me: *A Confederacy of Dunces*. It's absolutely brilliant and hilarious. It's also taken me six years to get around to reading it. Sorry, Chris.

6pm – Nap a bit more in the sunshine.

6.30pm – Waddle into the sea. The flan has now been digested so no risk of doing an egg sick in the waves.

7pm – Drip my way back to the sunbed. Perfect temperature now. Listen to a Billie Eilish album.

7.45pm – Feel guilty for not achieving anything today. Then I remember a funny book I was reading/writing told me to do nothing for a day and it gives me confidence to continue to do nothing much.

8:30pm – Get back home and decide to go for a sunset run. My favourite time of day for it. The sun is just disappearing off behind the mountains, and I feel like I'm in a movie starring myself. I then overthink it and start panicking that the movie would be boring and badly reviewed so I take my AirPods out and listen to nature to try to rid myself of a really annoying intrusive thought about a movie about me that would never be made.

9.15pm – Bella and my great pals Jenny and Alice cook a really nice dinner that we eat outside. Although all I can think about is getting it over with so I can gorge on cheese.

9.25pm – Begin gorging on cheese. Comte, Chaource, Boursin, Gruyère and my all-time favourite basic bitch cheese, Tartare (garlic and herb), were the order of the day. Tartare, by the way, is a French version of Boursin, which in itself is mad, but is even more delicious.

9.45pm – We found an old DVD of *Inspector Morse* so put on an episode of it. It was 1 hour 45 minutes long, fairly problematic in its treatment of the new female detective that joined the station, and weirdly seemed to forget to breadcrumb the actual murderer until the last five minutes. The flan and cheese made up for it. That was all washed down with a really nice local red wine from a town called Faugères.

Midnight (*minuit*) – As I've eaten quite a lot this evening, a good swig of Gaviscon is needed before bed. That's been the main difference between my twenties and thirties to be honest. Life is basically the same except there's a lot more heartburn medication in the house.

And that's that. That was my waste day. And it was fairly active. I'm not saying you have to sit still for the entire time, just don't worry about achieving anything other than eating a lot of dairy, laughing at a funny book then spending the day's final moments googling 'Jaguar Mark 2s' to see if I could afford a Morse car.

What's the Rush?

The person you are at ten or eleven might be the most you you'll ever be.

Thinking back to that time might be painful for you. I have to say it's a bit painful for me. At the time, I felt like an absolute weed. But as I've got older, I've realised that even though I didn't know who I was in the slightest, I was actually remarkably clear about who I wasn't. And more specifically, I knew inherently that my town's monthly underage disco, the Coconut Club, wasn't me in any way.

I spent my teenage years in Bishop's Stortford, which isn't a bad place. I don't think anyone would call it a great place either but I had a nice time. When I was there, it was very much an *Inbetweeners*-style town full of people that would like to think they were in *Skins* but were in no way cool enough. To bring it a little more up to date, Bishop's Stortford is Otis Milburn from *Sex Education* thinking he could get a part in *Euphoria*. I was Otis Milburn, I just didn't realise that. Sub-Otis actually, because at least he was interested in meeting and then, with a bit of luck, getting off with girls. I wouldn't have known what to do if confronted with Maeve Wiley. If I was 12 now, I wouldn't relate to any of those shows at all. I was more *Last of the Summer Wine*. I really loved *Last of the Summer Wine*. Maybe I've got it all wrong and age 11 isn't when I was the most me, instead I'll finally find my true self at 60.

I found this pursuit of working out how to be a teenager terrifying. My sister is ten years older than me, so from about eight onwards, I had the run of the place. It was the perfect set-up really. My sister, Catherine, is and always has been amazing. In my early years, she was the perfect grouchy, scary big-sister foil to me as the annoying little brother. I have great sympathy for her situation. There was suddenly a golden boy (with thick black hair) on the scene. Can you imagine how adorable I was at five? Catherine would have been fifteen and absolutely fuming that the family had been delivered a legend. But as we've grown up, I've valued our relationship so much. She is an immovable, supportive, brilliant, fun force in my life. Always on hand to help me with big adult decisions, calm in a crisis and a great sounding board when we're both rolling our eyes at the madness of our ageing parents. Someone to laugh at Mum and Dad with when they start worrying about where to park at something they're going to in two months' time. That said, she is still utterly terrifying if you cross her. When she went to university I was essentially able to behave like an only child, until it was time for me to go to university and sit around in halls myself eating Dairylea Dunkers for breakfast, lunch and dinner and pay nine grand a year for the privilege. Even more now. Thanks a lot, Nick Clegg.

Unlike a lot of my friends, it seemed, I really enjoyed hanging out with my parents. They were good at playing. They were both teachers, so they liked spending time with kids. And luckily, they *loved* spending time with us. They were both sporty so cricket, football, tennis, running, basketball and badminton were always on the agenda. Alongside that, gardening featured heavily. We didn't ever have the garden of my dreams (actual-cricket-ground size was the aim) but Bromley (long and thin), Epping (short and wide, full of moles) and then later on Bishop's Stortford (basically non-existent) provided a decent amount of weeds to help my mum shift. I also developed a fascination with lawnmowers. Yeah. Hard to make that sound cool, isn't it? I've certainly been selective with who I've told that to. Now I'm married, I'll happily put it in a book, but I'd still very much be a virgin if I'd led with this in my twenties. But that's who I am. Guys, I love grass. It's all connected with my love of cricket. I longed to mow a proper cricket pitch in the garden. The garden of our semi (lol) on Union Road in Bromley was the biggest, at 17 yards long. Five yards off a full-sized pitch. It had to do. I'd mow it, water it, use white emulsion paint to do the lines (Dad got cross at this) and even cover it with a shower curtain when it rained so I could get out there and play as soon as the clouds cleared.

Sport was a huge part of my childhood, as was videoing things. I was obsessed with special effects. I still am. I would make terrible little films with a Hi8 camcorder, which was the single most important thing I was ever given access to. I think my dad borrowed it from the school he was teaching at. He probably wasn't supposed to do that. But he's retired now and that job nearly killed him (more on that later), so what is anyone going to do? You can shove it up your arse. That little camera started my obsession with creating things and made me realise that making stuff was the most fun thing you could ever do. I'd shoot little videos of everything. From wholesome garden cricket matches (I'd later review the footage in slow motion to see if I had been out LBW), to the aforementioned special effects which often featured me setting fire to toy cars and simulating crashes. On one occasion, I made a life-sized model of myself using my own clothes stuffed with pillows and a papier mâché head which I then threw out of my bedroom window, filming it from two different angles. My mum was quite rightly furious with me because she thought it was actually me flying through the air. It was a great stunt, though. I do stand by that.

My passion for making videos naturally led to recording things on a microphone with a tape player and in turn that led me to radio, which became my obsession. I'd spend hours in my bedroom cueing up songs on Windows Media Player. The old old version of it meant you could have several windows open, so you could fire off jingles I'd stolen from Capital (boo) and Radio 1 as well as adding some funny sound effects up to the vocal. I know what you are thinking: *That's 'cool'*... Well, actually I do think that's quite cool. Not that I shouted about it to anyone back then. Being passionate about anything other than football and girls in early 2000s Bishop's Stortford would get you called 'GAY!' or 'PAEDO!' In hindsight, I'm so grateful I found a thing I truly loved. So, that's all I really cared about between the ages of 10 and 17. And how lucky I am to be currently living the life I was pretending to have when I was 12. Let's then ruin this lovely thought as we journey back in time to the Coconut Club.

Even thinking about the name of it makes me shudder. The Coconut Club was a nightclub experience set up for under-18s. Hell. Why was it even called that?! Bishop's Stortford isn't famous for coconuts. It's not particularly famous for anything last time I checked. Hang on, let me consult the internet ... Oh, actually,

Charli XCX went to the private school in the town. That's pretty cool. I didn't know that. I guess if you're Charli XCX you keep your Bishop's Stortford connection fairly quiet considering it's the least BRAT place imaginable. I wouldn't know whether the Coconut Club was BRAT, mainly because I never went. It might have been. Maybe it was BRAT not to go? Although I wouldn't have dreamt of saying it out loud, I found it very hard to conform to the idea that we all had to do the same thing at the same time. This wasn't a case of me being all cool and mysterious – I wasn't the moody, interesting outlier that everyone respected because he had even cooler things to do and was off writing poetry or painting. To be clear, I was at home watching wrestling videos. In hindsight, not BRAT. Every single time the Coconut rolled into town – I think once every couple of months – I just pretended I wasn't very well or that my mum and dad were taking us to visit Nan for the weekend. Basically I'd say or do anything to get out of going. I'd rather have been seriously ill in hospital than go and dance to Eiffel 65's 1990s megahit 'Blue (Da Ba Dee)' with some of the girls from the neigh-bouring school. The idea of dressing up in your finest Burton's shirt, boot-cut jeans and Lambretta trainers, a look only complete when accessorised with a Next bracelet, to go and 'pull' someone in a town hall in East Hertfordshire made me sad and anxious to my core. This wasn't snobbery by the way. I'd have *loved* to have had the confidence to relish this opportunity to show off to everyone and get off with a girl. Lord grant me the confidence of Matt Bruton on our Year 8 French exchange where he took things a little too literally and ended up exchanging saliva with the girl he was partnered up with. I was watching him do it. Not in a creepy way. Although this does now sound creepy. We were all on the coach ready to go and he was saying goodbye with his tongue and busy hands. I couldn't believe it. He was kissing a girl! I remember thinking that I would *never* be able to do that.*

Anyway, I never went to the god damn Coconut Club so to this day I still don't know exactly what was happening inside. I imagine it was like the Hacienda but instead of pill heads and stoners it was more Panda Pops and unwanted boners. My mates did go, however, and it was the *only* thing anyone could ever talk about. 'You going Coconut?' was said with the same sincerity that my friends now say, 'You going Glastonbury?' Perhaps the Coconut Club was amazing. Maybe I'm boring and I completely missed out. Maybe I should have gone once even if just to find the whole thing absurd and funny. Maybe everyone was just looking for something to do. Looking for somewhere to fit in. I wonder what percentage of the people who went genuinely loved it, though – 60 per cent? Maybe I'd still have been able to find strength in numbers being part of the 'anxious 40 per cent' nervously shuffling around the edge of the dancefloor as 'Brimful of Asha' was playing. I just saw it as something that was too 'grown up' for me at that time. I didn't want to speed through childhood. I was really enjoying the innocence of it all.

Meeting girls in general felt too grown up for me. I remember a couple of my friends chatting to some from nearby Hemel Hempstead on MSN Messenger and planning on getting the train to go and meet them one Saturday afternoon in real life. 'Hemel',

---

* NB: I have since managed to do that.

as those in the know call it, is only 30 miles away from Bishop's Stortford but I've just checked to see how long it would take to get there on the train and laughed out loud that on a bad day (which let's be honest is every day on our shit train network) it could take *two hours*. Bishop's Stortford to Tottenham Hale, Victoria line to Euston then a train out to Hemel. Unbelievably bleak. But to us at the time it was the MOST important and daring thing imaginable. And for me, my worst nightmare. My decision to avoid it at the time made me feel like the saddest dork to ever set foot on planet Earth, but with the benefit of hindsight, it was perhaps the greatest call of all time. 'What will you do when you get there?' I typed out on MSN. 'Dunno. Just walk around a bit. Maybe go cinema,' was the reply. Can you imagine the horror?! Well, yeah, you probably can. You probably lived this too. I bet you've got your very own Hemel Hempstead, haven't you? Will and Jack (yes, I'm shaming you both in print), returned with exotic stories about how they pulled the girls at the station after putting in the hard yards with a steamy afternoon of sitting down in silence at Cineworld watching the 1999 classic, *Stuart Little* (a solid film). I sort of wanted to do something like that myself because I knew it was the cool thing to do, but it just felt impossibly adult and scary and I couldn't face it. In reality, when they were telling me about it, although I felt left out, it did sound dreadful. And I was fine. You can duck out of something and just not do it if you don't want to. And you won't die. You might miss out, but ultimately I didn't have to do a four-hour round trip for a toothy snog and instead I sat at home and watched pirated episodes of *South Park*. I often chose the second option, and was happier for it.

In writing these memories down for the first time, I've real-ised I was probably quite an anxious child. And although I feel a little bit sad that I didn't really understand myself, I think that's a good thing. For one, confident 12-year-olds tend to be unbear-able pricks. Why are you so sure of yourself? What have you got to show off about? A tiny cock and some new shin pads? Get over yourself, Dean. I also don't think it was full-blown anxiety; I think it was just shyness and a tendency to overthink. It certainly wasn't crippling. I still feel like that boy from time to time. Sometimes I feel like I'm still not adult enough, particularly when I'm at a big party or event where everyone else seems to have their shit together. I can feel like that when I have to entertain famous, cool movie stars on the radio. Sometimes I don't feel cool and interest-ing enough for some of them and I have to really fight to not go into my shell and figuratively retreat into my bedroom and play *GTA* on the PlayStation. I don't, because the difference between childhood and adulthood is that, sometimes, you have to go to Hemel and pretend you know what you're doing. But remember, you can always go home and hang out with your dog afterwards.

I suppose you could say that I am, and always have been, sensi-tive to the world around me. For a few years at school I used to have 'funny turns' in lessons where suddenly everything would get muffled and loud and I'd hear my heartbeat incredibly loudly in my ears and my vision would shrink. I've never told anyone about this before because it sounds odd even now, but I've since realised that these were probably panic or anxiety attacks. Luckily I grew out of them (except when I'm really tired and stressed) but for a while I did think there was something wrong with me. Being a kid's hard, isn't it? Everyone does it at different speeds. Some of us are raring to get off with girls/boys and some of us are still playing with remote-controlled cars. The dream would have been both. I'm living that now. Well, not the boys bit as of yet.

Mostly, I did have a really nice time. I was happy faffing about with my computer, listening to music, making videos, listening to the radio and tinkering with electric train sets. I wasn't ready to give up being a 12-year-old. I suppose I felt like I had lots of growing to do before I was ready for the real world. And even as adults, it might not feel like it but we are all allowed to go at our own speed. Incidentally, the Coconut Club was held at a venue called the Rhodes Centre, after the famous colonialist Cecil Rhodes. The name has now been changed. See, I told you it was bad vibes.

A Quick List of Other Things I'm Forced to Like

The Coconut Club isn't the only thing I was told I had to be into:

* Sheep. I love animals but sheep have demonic eyes and I'm scared of them. They know things.
* Football. Gun to my head, if football didn't exist, I wouldn't give a shit.
* Marvel films. I hate that they pay the biggest actors in the world then paint them blue. You don't even know who's who.
* Tea. It tastes of nothing. Tea isn't a culture. Or a personality.
* Theme parks. Specifically rollercoasters. The ultimate in forced fun. Queuing for hours, everyone overreacting and screaming and all you do is sit there and feel sick. They're also dangerous and go wrong way too often.
* Cats. They hate us. Just accept it.
* Motorbikes. They sound like farts when they're revved.
* Quiz shows. So tedious. Why do I want to watch someone I don't know do a televised exam?
* TikToks where they stop people in the street. 'What song you listening to?!' FUCK OFF, MATE.
* Aubergines. They give me the creeps. Big, fleshy, sloppy blobs of gunk. Baba ganoush gets a pass.

*   The All on the Board thing at Tube stations. Fun when it started – it's just got a bit knowing and cynical now.
*   Parkrun. Love the idea of finding friends and community but ... No talking and running. Ever. It's a solo activity.
*   Skiing. Snow – great, cheese – fantastic, views – beautiful, sport – up for it. But ... I can't shake the idea that this is just a thing rich people invented to get away from the riffraff. Also, I couldn't do a week anywhere where hordes of men in gilets are there talking about investments.
*   Craft beer. Too fussy, too much of a 'scene'. All of it looks like dehydrated piss and most of it tastes like that too.
*   Padel. The game I actually like, but again it's been overrun by the gilet brigade. It feels like squash for the Steven Bartlett generation.

Radio Car Car

Driving a car was the main reason I wanted to be a grown-up. All I ever wanted to do was drive. I remember being on holiday in Sardinia when I was about 15 and my dad let me drive the hire car around a car park near the villa and I was so excited by it, I got an erection. I've never told anyone that. And I'm deeply sorry to all of you and everyone who knows me. Particularly my parents, who had to drive that Seat Alhambra (!) for the rest of the holiday. Cars were (clearly) a very early passion of mine. I firmly believe that being able to drive is the best thing about becoming an adult. Thanks to some grainy photographs of my early years, it's apparent that all I've wanted to do is be behind the wheel of something. On my 18th birthday, my mum presented me with a collage of photos of me in various vehicles. There was a milk float, a fire engine, dodgems, bumper boats and my favourite method of transport when I was four – a small blue pedal tractor that I used to attach a trailer to so I could help Mum transport things around the garden. God I miss that thing. It feels very gender typical of me to love cars, doesn't it? But it wasn't like I grew up the son of a racing driver or anything. Or even had parents that particularly loved cars. I instinctively just did.

I grew up in a really exciting time for cars. Seat Alhambras aside, the 1980s and 1990s into the 2000s produced some of the all-time greats. It was the era when the technology that is commonplace now was just starting to be introduced into what was quite an analogue era. It was a time when electric windows were exciting and luxurious. Automatics were seen as futuristic and power steering made you feel like Superman when trying to park in a tight spot. I loved the late 1990s/early 2000s rally cars. Big up the Subaru Impreza and the Toyota Celica in particular. I also really loved – even if I didn't fully understand what I was watching – Formula One. I thought it was amazing and ridiculous and obviously I lusted after the mad supercars of the era. The Ferrari F50 and the Jaguar XJ220 were my particular favourites. But truthfully, despite all these feats of modern engineering, I really *really* loved quite run-of-the-mill, ordinary (most would say boring) cars. Perhaps it was all I was exposed to. The first car I remember in the family was a silver B-reg Nissan Sunny. It was basically the same age as me but by the time I was ten it had already done well over 100,000 miles, which was way more than I'd done. And the little gem was still going, just about.

I think about that car a lot. It was the supporting character in a formative part of my childhood. And it's oddly central to why I am like I am and why I do what I do. For a brief bit of background, as teachers, Mum and (in particular) Dad moved schools fairly regularly. This often meant we'd have to up sticks and relocate nearer to wherever his new school was. Obviously this was far from easy to coordinate for my parents, and there were weird times when Mum was teaching at a school close to where we used to live and had to go back there every day, or Dad would have to get up at 5am and commute, or sometimes I'd have to stay with friends after school to avoid a long journey. There was one period of my life when I was still at primary school in Bromley, in Kent, my mum was teaching at a secondary school a few miles away but my dad had taken a new job north of London in Enfield. We'd decided to move to Essex. I'm not sure why. In hindsight, I'm not sure they do either. I assumed my parents had everything sorted when I was a kid. I assume Essex happened because they were probably stressed and just wanted to find a nice place for us all to live. So we lived there. And for a year or so, as Dad was dashing off to Enfield, Mum and I would bundle into the Sunny at just before 7am and start the 90-minute, 60-mile journey around the M25 to the opposite end of London. It's mad when I think about it now. But these bits of family madness are commonplace. The sacrifices parents make to minimise the disruption for their kids never ceases to amaze me; they made their lives difficult just to minimise the upheaval for us. They obviously didn't *want* us to have to move so often and have to deal with the disruption and baldness-inducing stress that brings, but that's life. And jobs. And families. You just have to get on with it. It's only really looking back, now that I've moved a few times, held down a job, tried to build a network of friends, find a partner and find my place in the world that I truly realise just how much they did for me and my sister while also trying to progress their own lives too.

That journey to school, as well as being quite a slog, was where Mum and I became a great team. It would be too much to say I looked forward to those cold mornings where the car would barely sputter into life, but largely I do remember it being great fun. My parents *are* so much fun, which helped, and they loved an adventure. And that's what it was sold to me as. And to this day, I love going on road trips and adventures of my own. Mum made it feel exciting. We'd have a weekly routine where if I had a club to go to or she had to stay and referee a netball match or something, she'd arrange for us to stay at one of her colleagues' houses. A lovely French teacher friend of hers called Francine was my favourite. Mainly because the spare room I stayed in was also the computer room of their house in Orpington and I could play games on it after I'd done my homework. But also there was always great cheese there. Because French. Otherwise, Mum would be waiting for me after school with something from her school's tuck shop in the glovebox. Fruit Gums were always crowd-pleasers and would last ages. We'd then set off on the motorway and if I was lucky, we'd have McDonald's as a treat when I'd just done cricket practice and we wouldn't be home in time for her to make dinner.

The other really magical bit of this part of my life was that it was when I was properly exposed to radio. Hours of it. And it was breakfast radio. I've since realised after a few hundred therapy sessions and the odd interview about my career, that the AM radio (google it if you're under 30) of that Nissan Sunny sealed my fate and set me well and truly on the path to becoming a radio anorak. We'd have the *Virgin Radio Breakfast Show* on every morning. I hadn't a clue what Radio 1 was by this point – sorry, big bosses. Virgin, because it was broadcast on medium wave, was all the car could get. 1215 AM was the frequency. And the sound quality was obviously rubbish. For a modern comparison for those not ancient like me, it sounded like an AirPod if you'd accidentally put it through the wash. But I loved how their breakfast show sounded.

It was hosted by Russ Williams and Jono Coleman. *Russ & Jono* was the show's imaginative name and it just sounded fun. In fact, I've since nicked a couple of their features. One of them was where they'd get actual listeners into the studio on a Friday morning and I turned it into 'Feet Up Friday' for years when I was on afternoons on Radio 1. It's a great, simple trick to make the show sound full of energy and demonstrate that people actually wanted to hang out with you. The real trick with entertainment radio is making sure you hear as many listeners as possible. Not only does it make the show sound big, it encourages other listeners to take part too. If you hear someone doing something funny and it makes everyone laugh, that's infectious. Also, if you hear people that you relate to, you want to come back and hang out again and again. And I did! The music was also great. It was the early 1990s so it was a soundtrack of Oasis, Blur and Alanis Morissette. A *lot* of Alanis Morisette. Mum and I still recite the lyrics to 'Hand in My Pocket' to each other every now and then. 'I've got one hand in my pocket ... the other's giving a V sign!' This was my first introduction to swearing with your hands. Thanks, Russ and Jono! I do remember one slightly awkward moment when a caller on their show started talking about how winning a competition that morning felt 'orgasmic'. I asked my mum what that was. She didn't really have an answer. When I eventually did piece it together several years later, I assumed that her lack of explanation was due more to British awkwardness than it was any comment on her own experience with Dad. I'm appalled that line came into my head.

Obviously at the time I didn't think, *Oh wow, I love that radio soundtracks people's days and seeps in without them realising it, playing the perfect song at the perfect time.* Mainly because it seeped in without me realising it. But I now work in radio and have studied it for many years, so I've had time to work out exactly why I love it. And this early memory sums it all up perfectly. Radio works brilliantly because it's always there. It's reliable and if it's also good, it should elevate your day and add to it. I'm not saying it is necessarily life-changing but I definitely think it can be life-enhancing. It's designed to bring people together, to form a community, to offer its listeners a friend or companion. It was always the thing I took with me wherever I went – it still is. Moving schools often, my one constant pal was the radio and I'd set up my Sony hi-fi system with a CD multi-changer and separate speakers in my bedroom as soon as we moved into each new house. When the time came for me to go to university, my very first task as I unpacked my life, this time into halls, was to set up the very same (by this point retro) hi-fi. I was a mad Radio 1 fan by then so I couldn't wait to have them soundtrack this exciting part of my life. I'd been tipped off by some mates who listened to Chris Moyles on the way home from school and I was hooked. I then discovered Scott Mills on early breakfast and I was in. I'd wake up extra early just to catch the last bit of Scott's show before I had to get ready. When I started university in September 2004, I was keen to make sure Moyles, Jo Whiley, Colin and Edith, Scott and Zane Lowe were with me. That was a legendary line-up. And bizarrely, one that I would slot into just three years later, which slightly blows my mind thinking about it now. In my university days, I would sometimes catch a bit of Moyles but obviously as a student, I'd get up quite late, usually just in time for Jo and her Live Lounge, which was well on its way to becoming the global phenomenon it is now and long before it was copied by every other media outlet. It felt like the biggest artists in the world were queueing up around the block to be on with her. Then came Colin and Edith for a slightly ruder, more studenty type of show, which I loved, and then I'd always try to catch Scott. He was consistently funny, daring and so creative. I loved the games and the features and the spontaneity of it. It was so, so good. The day would be rounded off by the king of new music – Zane Lowe. That show single-handedly changed my music taste. He introduced me to The Killers, Arctic Monkeys, Adele, Kanye West, Future Heads and Kings of Leon, along with countless indie bands that I became obsessed with. To this day, I still adore Maxïmo Park. I'd die for that band. I was playing them on student radio and then I'd listen to Zane and get such a buzz from him also championing them. It was such an exciting show, with the biggest interviews and 'The Hottest Record in the World'; every night, everyone in our flat would be in the kitchen making a terrible dinner, probably consisting of beans, and *had* to listen.

As well as those must-listen moments, radio often has a more metronomic and workhorse-like duty to fulfil. From my GCSEs onwards, I would leave the radio on in my bedroom when I went off to do an exam because there was great comfort in knowing that it was going to still be there chattering away when I got back. Walking back into the room and hearing that it was still burbling away, no matter what's going on in the world, made me feel calm and reminded me that there was more to life than maths exams. It's a great reminder that the world will always keep moving, that you're just a small part of it and therefore so is your stressful day. I still keep the radio on if I'm anxious about the day ahead. I was recently doing a screen test for a big TV show that I didn't really want to do but was flattered into it and was dreading. It felt like an exam and I felt like a teenager again so I left Classic FM on in my house because I wanted to come home and feel that calmness that I used to feel after an A level. Radio can be an amazing constant in your life; it always has been in mine. And I find it's very rarely the 'big' moments that stick with you. I often remind myself of this. It doesn't have to be an interview with a big star or a huge stunt that runs over a week or so – the joy is in the consistency. The daily conversation with listeners, a stupid sound effect, a great caller or just a genuinely funny slip-up. The little bits make up the whole. There's a lesson in that, isn't there? I remember Scott Mills dedicating Nelly's 'Hot In Herre' to me while I was delivering pizzas, I remember hearing Ludovico Einaudi for the first time on Classic FM while I was revising for my A levels and I remember Chris Moyles's sports presenter, the great Juliette Ferrington, saying the words 'sausage party' for some reason and that becoming a clip he used for years. I'd always laugh when he did. After writing this chapter, I called up my mum to reminisce about that period of our lives, and she remembered all the silly little bits too. Without prompting she mentioned Francine who we stayed with, McDonald's after cricket and the Nissan Sunny. I mentioned the sweets in the glovebox and she laughed and said, 'I can't believe we did that for so long. How mad!'

I'm probably not going to be a parent – and by the way, I'm really OK with that. But I would urge you now, if you are one, to give yourself a break. And to remember that it's often the little, unexciting things that can become your child's happiest memories. The vast expanses of time with them, the routine, the seemingly mundane moments: they all contain pockets of magic. I don't remember what I got for any of my Christmases at that age but I do remember the daily Fruit Gums and long meandering chats with my mum while listening to funny people on the radio. Just being there with them I think might well be the key to it all. Showing up. In those moments I felt loved, I felt safe, I felt happy. And reminiscing now, at the tender age of 800, makes me feel exactly the same. It's also served as a nice reminder that perhaps life isn't nearly as complicated as we make it.

School
Daze

'I didn't like school' is quite a common review, isn't it? Let me tell you this, though, you are not supposed to. You have to go to school EVERY day and you're there for SO long that it would be insane to like it all the time, or even most of the time. Life doesn't work like that. I couldn't get my head around it when I started school and it felt so unfair. For most of us, school was probably a mixed bag *at best*. I vividly remember, on my first day at big school, looking around at the brutish, sweaty, loud Year 11s and sixth formers who just felt impossibly old, fully grown adults and thinking, *Yeah, secondary school's not for me. There's no fucking way I'm going to be one of them in a few years, no thanks.* They were all dicks. It was another reason I just wanted to be 11 forever, thank you.

But, somehow, without you realising it, time at school passes absurdly quick, and suddenly you're sitting in a hot sports hall in June, sweating your fully descended balls off trying to recall the ins and outs of the Night of the Long Knives. Bizarre really. I never want to be one of those exhausting people in the public eye (nearly always men) who, come results day, decide to climb up on their high horse (that they bought with money they made themselves with help from nobody, *especially* their teachers who wrote them off) and rush to social media to tell you about the exams they failed and despite that insist on bragging about how great their life is, and proclaiming how they didn't need exams or teachers or anyone or anything. 'I didn't even have shoes! Or water! Or air! We couldn't even afford air when I was a kid! And look at me now!' they brag, 'I'm a fucking millionaire!' Those people should be forced to take a GCSE in learning how not to become pricks; I'd be happy to mark the papers. No, I don't want to be one of those blokes, but each to their own. Exams aren't for everyone. Formal education isn't for everyone. But it is for some – some are great at it. And to rubbish the entire system is an insult to those that did well. So shut your stupid face, Lord Sugar.

Anyway, exams! I wasn't brilliant at them but I did have shoes, water, air and with some good old-fashioned hard work, some amazing teachers and some dedicated parents I managed to do well. But it didn't come naturally to me. Learning facts, remembering them and writing them down under time pressure like it's one of those boring, overcomplicated BBC One daytime quiz shows was insane to me. And it was far from the best way for me to actually *learn*, which let's not forget is supposed to be the point of school. In general, though, I did enjoy trying my best even when the lessons didn't make a great deal of sense. English, languages, geography and history were my strongest subjects. English was definitely my favourite. That's thanks to my parents reading to me and making up stories. I came alive when I was reading aloud in lessons, I loved writing essays about Atticus Finch in *To Kill a Mockingbird* or trying to get my head around Shakespeare's batshittery. I have also always loved playing around with words. Like batshittery.

I also loved history. My eyes lit up when we learnt about the Russian maniacs of the early nineteenth century. What came before us is still really interesting to me. It's why we're all doing what we're doing. I was just as fascinated by geography. Why is the world like it is? Why does it rain? What the fuck is a volcano? Soil! It's genuinely interesting to me because we all came from it. And we shall return there too. Oh, and why foreign languages? Because a basic grasp of French will serve me well when I settle down in Paris with my third wife someday.

The other periods in my school timetable filled me with quite a lot of dread. I naturally veered towards the lighter, more humanitarian subjects. Science and maths I found tricky. They were too mysterious to me, which is odd considering they tend to deal with precision and fact-based conclusions. I just didn't get a lot of it. And I'm not proud of that. I wish my brain worked better in that world but I'd be sitting there thinking, *WHY ARE YOU TELLING ME ABOUT IRON?! And why is that different from an ION?!* Lessons on Fibonacci's triangle in maths might just as well have been someone standing up at the front doing farts for an hour. I'd have understood that way more. Here's the thing, though: it's OK not to get everything. No one told me that at school. You were expected to just understand all of it. And all grasp it at the same time and to the same level. That's impossible. And unfair. I was lucky that I wasn't thick and had some inter-est in, and even passion for, certain subjects. That carried me through until I was eventually allowed to leave. But I can totally see why kids are turned off by school. You're herded through largely same system. Millions of different brains and person-alities all forced through one small learning funnel. There has to be a better way.

I was dreadful at pressurised exams; I know that plenty of people are – so why are the tests standardised? What is that teaching you? All I learnt was how to be anxious and sad. I still have nightmares about my A levels. I fucking hated every second of those exams. Coursework, fieldwork, practicals and performances are all brilliant, sign me up! But I still fail to understand the benefit of being made to sit down for two hours to try to recall the details of Charles I's life. All I remember was writing about his execution while quietly hoping that my own head would fall off so I'd have an excuse to leave.

I don't come bearing solutions, sadly. It's a very difficult problem to fix, but there's no way every single child can be expected to learn in the exact same way. There's also no easy way around having to learn the basics. You just should have to do that bit. You have to learn numbers. You have to learn letters. You have to learn how science works and how we all coexist and how life is made. But aside from that, maybe you should be allowed to pick. Not just the subjects, but the areas too? If I was prime minister (could happen), I would suggest new lessons for all secondary schools. I'm amazed that no one teaches us about money management, for example. Tax! No one teaches us about tax! Why not?! Rent! Mortgages! What the fuck is a mortgage?! I still don't know and I've got a crippling one. Hedge funds! Pensions! Insurance! Tell us about these things!

Basic politics and media should be compulsory from an early age. I know these subjects that are taught more widely now at GCSE but that's only a recent change. It was only ever an option at A level when I was a spotty, lanky freak. And let's not forget that A levels are exams you take at an age when you're already allowed to vote and you are no longer legally required to still be in formal education, so only a tiny number of people would ever be taught about them. Politics, which is simply the way our country operates, is fundamental to the rest of our lives. Why was I sitting around learning about oxbow lakes when I should also have been told about who owns the newspapers in the UK and why that's important? We should be taught about the big corporations that don't pay tax. Teachers should be alerting us to mad world leaders being racist. This is embarrassing to say but I didn't truly understand the role of right-wing newspapers until I worked in WHSmith when I was 16 and a very smart manager pointed out that essentially each tabloid and broadsheet had vested interests that therefore dictated its editorial content. Smith's in Bishop's Stortford taught me more about Rupert Murdoch than school did. Now that's a legacy.

We should be taught about privilege. We should be made aware of our *own* privilege. Whatever school you're at, you should be told about all the other ones. I had no idea about Eton and Harrow. I didn't even really understand the advantage kids who went to private school would have over me throughout my life. I didn't know what a boarding school was like. I mean, I read Harry Potter but to my knowledge even the posh lot over at Marlborough didn't have owls. Similarly, most kids don't have a frame of reference for schools that were less well off than theirs. I sort of did with my parents because my mum taught at a private girl's school for a while and my dad at a pretty challenging comprehensive in Enfield. I was lucky in that respect because I could see that The

Bishop's Stortford High School sat squarely in the middle of those two. Devastatingly, I didn't truly understand racism and the privilege I had as a straight white man from the south until I was in my twenties. That's awful. Yes, it's partly my fault – and my privilege – but surely this idea should have at least been mentioned to me at school. I hope it's now at least part of the conversation, if not the syllabus. It must be insanely difficult to be a teenager in 2025 with the pressures of being constantly online and 'gettable'. I certainly benefitted from a more analogue adolescence, but I can't help but feel a little jealous that the huge benefit of the world's discourses and resources are all contained in your phone. It's wonderful that you can watch and read smart takes on current global events, discover essays from people much smarter than you about the subjects you're studying to help broaden your knowledge and have access to every documentary ever made to aid your learning. Not only this, you can connect to people from other parts of the world in a way I just couldn't at school. For example, a TikTok-ker showing you what life in Ukraine during the current conflict with Russia is like could provide an obviously devastating but nonetheless up-to-date eyewitness account, which in turn could add to your understanding of Stalinist Russia. Time travel is basically now as real as we can get it! My point being, I would have been able to gear my studies much more to my needs and interests if I'd had more than just Microsoft Encarta at my fingertips.

So what's the point of it then? The grades might be important to 'get you to the next stage' but they largely don't ever get talked about again; however, school is great for other things. It ushers you through the most difficult, most hormonal years of your life.

It gives you a structure when you're at your most foolish and frontal lobe-less. You know, those years when you think it's a good idea to chokeslam your friends into a pile of bags at the bus stop. Speaking of which, it also socialises you. It can give you friends for life and it also teaches you how to put up with and work alongside people you might hate. It gives you the opportunity to work out what you like and dislike and maybe, if you're lucky, it'll help you discover a passion. School humbles and hardens you. You should feel deeply embarrassed about how you behaved, looked and acted sometimes and take comfort that you'll hopefully never be as awkward and gawky again. You'll never have to eat school dinners again. Unless you're a teacher. Oh, and once you leave, it spells the end of sitting exams on things you don't give a shit about. I still think the worst memories I have in my life aren't of people I love dying or heartbreaks; they're of sitting there staring down the barrel of a two-hour non-calculator maths GCSE paper wishing I was dead.

Every single one of us will have had to do at least 12 years of school, and while primary school is pretty much just a place to make dreadful pasta art that your parents still keep on the fridge 20 years later, secondary school is where things get difficult. While there are many objectionable things about the education system, like having to learn a bunch of things you'll never need to use in your life (long division for starters, that can get to fuck), it does offer one brilliant thing. School is a glorious and brief moment in life where you have the chance to see your mates *every single day*. You don't realise how lucky you are to get to hang out with your friends all the time until you're an adult and working in an office with people you'd never willingly be seen dead hanging out with at the pub. It's even better if you unite and have a common enemy to rail against – that enemy is the school, by the way. Friends make it all just about bearable.

Greggy
No Mates

I am cross with myself this morning. Cross and disappointed. I spent last night with one of my oldest friends and it was as brilliant as it always is when we hang out. I laughed for hours just like we had the last time we saw each other eight months ago. Eight months. That's not OK. We live a 27-minute train journey away from each other in the same city. There's something going wrong with us here. I bet you're nodding right now because you've had a similar experience, haven't you?

Pat and I immediately became best mates on day one of university and I knew this was going to happen within the first ten seconds of meeting him. We did the same English and drama course and early on in freshers' week there was an induction where we'd meet the 40 other drama luvvies with whom we'd be spending the next three years. *Whom* is a funny word, isn't it. WHOOOOOOM. In any group of 40 people, the chances of you liking all of them to the same degree is *very* slight. The chances of being in a group of 40 eighteen-year-olds studying drama and liking every single one of *them* is zero. The heady mixture of new-term anxiety and overconfidence emanating from the drama studio made me feel like I was an unwitting contestant on the first episode of a reality show. I immediately wanted to pack up my things, move to Cambodia and enrol in a university there to study geography. It was overwhelming and I immediately became shy Greg again.

The first day of the course was predictably intense and drama-y, full of over-the-top warm-ups, trust exercises, standing up and telling everyone who you are and saying three quirky things every-one needed to know about you. The most common answers were 'I'm pretty messy!' or 'I'm so disorganised lol!' or 'I'm always late for things!' I was sitting next to Pat as the fifth person said, 'I'm quite untidy to be honest', and he whispered to me, 'I want to kill these people.' That was all I needed. He was my guy. We were inseparable for the next three years.

I remember we peeled off from a freshers' event to go to his halls to carry on drinking there and as I went into his room and sat down on the bed, he handed me a Bible and very earnestly said, 'Shall we read a verse aloud to each other?' I laughed nervously, thinking that I'd made a huge mistake, and perhaps he wasn't my guy after all. He was God's guy. 'Open it,' he said. I obliged and immediately burst out laughing when I saw that he'd hollowed out the pages to make a perfect safe storage area for some weed. We sat around smoking, drinking and listening to old comedy albums as if we were at university in 1970. I wish I'd been at university in 1970. We listened to hours of Peter Cook sketches and basically became best mates in the space of three days. Over the next three years, that friendship helped me grow immeasurably; I found someone who indulged my passion for funny things. We were always being silly – doing stupid voices, coming up with characters and daft 'bits' – but we also bizarrely realised that we both had girlfriends we wanted to break up with who happened to be at the same university in

London. And there we were, one gloomy weekday in October, sitting next to each other on an Anglia Railways train to go and do the deed. We were both really sad but so relieved and, looking back now, reliant on each other's slightly buttoned-up emotions to find the confidence to do it. We felt like massive shits on that train together back to Norwich but we knew it was the right thing. Reading this now, you might think it was a heartless thing to do, but we were both stupid 18-year-olds and it was better for both girls involved that they had nothing to do with us. They dodged two idiotic bullets. Pat has since gone on to become a successful and incredibly well-respected comedian and an obscenely talented model maker but back then – along with someone else who went on to great things in the alternative comedy world, John Kearns – we would put on comedy nights, do plays together and they'd often join me on my student radio shows as we came up with stupid ideas like sending John into the cinema in town to do live film reviews. Still a great idea, that. Maybe I'll bring it back. I just remember it as a really fun, creative, silly time where we were all just dicking about without a care in the world. Heaven. They were two amazing friends who arrived at just the right time to help me along the way to working out who I was. I love being around really funny people. The type of funny that makes your face ache with just a look – and there isn't anyone funnier than those two. I feel like that excited 18-year-old every time we hang out, so why doesn't it happen more often?

The easy, boring cop-out answer is: 'Life' – but what does that mean? Everyone's busy, everyone's tired and everyone's stressed. These are all givens but I bet I'd feel better stealing even half an hour with a good mate, and I'd certainly be better off doing that than sitting like a moron scrolling on my phone. Yes, it's annoying to leave the house sometimes and travel miles and the sofa *is* very inviting, but some of the fondest memories of my life involve Pat and John and we just don't see each other enough. It was Pat's 40th birthday recently and John and I met him on a rainy Monday afternoon in Hammersmith because he'd booked something secret for us to do. He'd insisted on booking axe-throwing for three, at 4.20pm on a Monday. Already ridiculous. There was no one else in there apart from the instructor and a playlist of manly axe music (Muse, Royal Blood, Foo Fighters, Kasabian. Basically the Radio X playlist. Sorry, Radio Axe). We spent two hours pissing ourselves laughing that this was how he wanted to spend his 40th. It was perfect nonsense. By the end of it, we'd mastered some trick shots, made friends with the instructor and thrown more axes than a bunch of drunk Vikings after a day's pillaging. One of the main reasons we don't see each other much is that we're all fairly useless at planning. They also tend to work evenings and I'm up at 5am, but these things can be worked around. We should try to buck the trend because when we say 'life got in the way', we're wilfully ignoring the fact that friends *are* your life. When it's all said and done, your life will be judged not by how busy you were at work but by how many times you threw axes with your best mates in a weird cork-clad bar in Hammersmith.

Something I have fallen foul of is working too much. My problem is – and this won't garner much sympathy – that I take on too many projects because they're often incredibly fun and reward-ing. I'm not even talking about money here. I'm not particularly motivated by money but I'm easily flattered into something that sounds enjoyable because all I've ever wanted to do is fun things. What I don't realise is that by filling my days and evenings with work, I neglect my actual life and therefore my friends. The gaps between work should be the nourishing bits of real life, but I'm in a position where the lines are blurred and work becomes fun and fun becomes work. In reality, it's *all* work. It may be fun but it's not using the truly switched-off, pleasurable bit of my brain. I'm currently going through a bit of an audit on my work–life balance and even though it's beyond ironic that I'm sitting here at work writing a book, it's a very useful exercise to undertake.

There are other reasons why you can't maintain friendships quite as well as you used to when you get older. You might have a new baby, for example, you and your partner move in together and you rightly have to prioritise that a lot of the time, but the thing we don't talk about enough is perhaps you don't spend as much time with some of your friends because you just don't really like them anymore. It's completely OK for friendships to drift away from you, but that doesn't mean it isn't sad. It can be particularly upsetting because most of the time there isn't a moment where you declare the friendship over, there isn't the chance for a messy break-up or a big final fight or that devastatingly sad evening where you exchange the belongings that you kept in each other's flats. Christ that's a bleak episode, isn't it? I'll never forget those moments. In my memory it was always raining and always cold and dark and often a flatmate (or even worse, a parent) was used as the intermediary as you meekly handed back a lamp or their favourite Bon Iver vinyl.

In a good friendship, both sides need to be engaged; if there's an imbalance it's exhausting, and being friends with someone should never be that. I have found this very hard to get my head around. None of this stuff is easy, and if you're a nostalgist like me, letting go of friendships that perhaps used to be very close but don't nourish you both anymore is tough. I've sometimes found myself being the one that's constantly offering up dates, suggesting ideas and activities and getting nothing back. I've caught this imbalance and taken a step back and if they pop up and suggest something, then fantastic. But if there's radio silence, I'd suggest that it might be time to reconsider what the friendship even is. Sometimes friendships just fizzle out, and it can be no one's fault in particular but once you've come to terms with it, you can really focus on the new ones you've made and the special ones you're left with. You don't have to be dramatic about it all (it shouldn't end up as a *Game of Thrones*-style Red Wedding) but it's a useful exercise to take a step back and work out where all your friends are in the league. It's normal for friends to go up and down the table. Some are promoted, some lose form and drop down a bit, others put in loads of effort and climb up and some are relegated forever. They might spend a few years in the lower leagues and realise they shouldn't have let it slip and claw their way back to the top flight, but that's on them. If you don't like the football analogy and prefer a bit of politics, look at it this way: you're the prime minister of your own life and it's good to work out who's in your cabinet to help you govern effectively. It could well be time for a cabinet reshuffle – someone who's been slacking as your Chancellor of the Exchequer might need to be demoted to Secretary of State for Work and Pensions. Still an important role but no longer the number two. It's also worth checking that you've given each other positions of similar standing. There's no point making someone your foreign secretary if they see you as more of a Minister for Transport. Sometimes, in severe cases, certain friends may have brought the government into disrepute and they need to be sacked. It will hopefully never come to that but you have to be prepared. I've done it once in my life and it wasn't great but it was for the best. Believe me, he's better off on the back benches.

The world is a fucking bin fire at times, so having good friends that enhance your life and don't sap energy from it is crucial. You don't have to inform your friends of their demotion or promotion, by the way; their roles will just change as you move forward. As I mentioned earlier, the main joy of school is that you get to hang out with your mates automatically without having to plan it. You're there spending whole days together, week in, week out. You're completely spoilt by this when you're a kid and you don't think it'll ever change. It's only later in life you start appreciating just how free, easy and spontaneous life used to be. There was a bizarre amount of free time. Whole days would just float by and the only thing you'd need to do was wander around town, decide to go bowling, sit in Pizza Hut for a couple of hours nailing the all-you-can eat buffet, head to the park, then go and play football, and finally sit around watching wrestling and then moronically run people over on *Grand Theft Auto*. It was bliss.

We moved to Bishop's Stortford when I was about 14, and very fortunately we lived just two roads away from the cricket club. It was and still is an amazing part of town. My mates and I would spend all day down there in the summer holidays. There would just be a revolving door of people coming along and bowling for a bit, going up to the bar to get a Coke and some crisps (usually Frazzles), then getting padded up and hitting the ball as far as possible. Afterwards, we might mix it up with some tennis on the nearby courts, and when we got older, we'd graduate to a pub trip in the evening – armed with our fake IDs. Every single town has a pub which the teenagers know are lax about ID and for us the Robin Hood was always the easiest one to get into. By the time we were of driving age, we used to suggest a trip to Harlow dog track or the enormous all-you-can-eat Chinese on the way to Colchester. We were so lucky to have all that free time to mooch about. There were four of us that would do everything together. *All the time.* This is why *The Inbetweeners* resonated so much when it came out. We're all still mates, I'm happy to report. From that four, Will is my absolute best mate in the world – more of a brother really – and yet even with him, there's that adult distance. He's someone I used to see every single day for *hours* on end, but adulthood means that the periods of time between seeing each other are longer. Each catch-up is now front-loaded with the obligatory half an hour of 'How are you?', 'How's work, etc.', 'How's being a dad?' The response is often, '*How long you got?*' whereas teenage friendships are just continuous – you never have to reintroduce yourself or catch up on life, it just carries on as part of your gloriously simple routine, your lives intertwined. Wake up, brush your teeth, have breakfast, see your mates. But now, in our adult lives, there are about 45 things between breakfast and seeing your mates.

All the best for the future

I think I've found a good solution to a few of these problems, though. Introducing 'the eight-minute phone call'! I read about it in the *New York Times* – because I'm very smart – and I think it's a completely brilliant idea. It's perfect for busy adults who can't synchronise diaries without ending up saying things like, 'I can't make September, I'm training for a marathon, what about December?' 'Oh, that's no good, I'm in Stoke for a conference ...' Blah blah, boring, shut up. In the article, the journalist Jancee Dunn quotes a Harvard professor by the name of Dr Bob Waldinger (FANTASTIC name, by the way. It's a WALDINGER of a name) who states that most busy people 'tend to think that in some unspecified future, we'll have a "time surplus" where we'll be able to connect with old friends ... That may never materialize, so pick up the phone and invest the time right now.' He's right, isn't he? There's no set way to do the eight-minute phone call and it doesn't even need to be eight minutes precisely. Maybe start with eight and then see how it all goes if you're having a nice time. Do 10! 20! 30! Whatever, just maybe give it a go – but sell it to your friend by explaining that you've just read the legendary Greg James's book and he told you to do it (after he nicked it from a much smarter and better writer who doesn't keep on doing annoying asides). You can maybe do it more regularly, too, over the course of a couple of weeks or so, depending on how much depth you want to go into. The content is for you to decide! Sometimes it could be the functional 'How are you?', 'How's work?' stuff which means that it's out of the way by the time you get to the pub for that long overdue face-to-face, but also it could just be mindless ramblings about the latest episode of

Married at First Sight or – let's get real here – who you've shagged and/or who you want to shag. Eight minutes of pure base-level gossip. There's a podcast in that … No! No more podcasts, Greg! Be strict with the timings by having a 'hard out' on the call. My good friend and co-conspirator Alice Levine calls them 'transitionals'. Conversations when she's on the way to something, thus giving a time limit on the chat. She's very open about it and states 'THIS IS A TRANSITIONAL' at the start of the call. And I respect the madness. That way, you'll both know where you stand, and I think you'll be surprised at the amount of ground you can cover in that time. It's the perfect workaround if you are genuinely too busy and stressed out to talk for longer or meet up. We should deploy this idea with the understanding that if 'too busy' actually means 'slumped on the sofa watching a Glenn Powell film', then arrange that eight-minute phone call.

Oh, and while you're slumped around on the sofa trying to work out if he's been created by AI – I think he might have been – you'll no doubt be engrossed in multiple WhatsApp groups and up to your eyeballs in memes. I love nothing more than a load of mad, inappropriate group chats and WhatsApp is undoubtedly really fun and a great way to stay in touch with people, but let's not try to convince ourselves that it's anywhere near as valuable as some real one-on-one time together. Sharing a meme shows you're thinking of someone, but speaking to or seeing them shows you really care. I really loved the landline call when I was much younger. I'd call up Will for a chat on his house phone (I still remember the number but for obvious reasons can't print it) and the *horror* if a parent answered! Cause of death? Will's mum picked up the phone. I also loved the joy of having a cordless phone which meant you could go to your bedroom and chat to your mates for hours like you'd seen on American TV shows. I felt like *Clarissa Explains It All* or *Blossom*. Before I get too lost in nostalgia that younger readers will no doubt have to google, make the call, recapture the teenage spontaneity ... for *at least* eight minutes. Anything less is basically a cold call from an energy provider.

Shove It Up Your Class

I grew up for the first bit of my life in Bromley in Kent, or as some people try to claim, London. It's not really London. At a push, it's Greater London but there's nothing particularly great about it. Having said that, the aforementioned David Bowie is from there. Emma Raducanu grew up there too and so did the comedian Rob Beckett. In fact, I used to sound a bit like Rob Beckett when I was a kid. I went to Raglan Primary, on Raglan Road, and my mum still has a video of me at a harvest festival where we were all assigned a vegetable and because I was tall, I was given a large one. An absolutely enormous marrow. For some reason you had to stand up, hold it above your head and shout out what you had and what colour it was. My turn came and I stood up proudly, pressed it above my head and bellowed:

'A MARRA IS GREEEEEYN!'

I honestly sounded like an East End greengrocer. I find accents absolutely fascinating – I always have – and I love messing around with them. Anyone who listens to my radio show will attest to this. I'd actually like to still have the accent I had when I was six, but where did it go? Moving around so much as a kid might have had something to do with it, I suppose. I lived in fairly nondescript places, each with a variation on a London/Essex/Kent accent, known as the Estuary English accent. Lots of the kids I grew up with sounded like either Rob Beckett or Stacey Solomon.

Somehow over time, though, I have ended up with a sort of vaguely well-spoken southern accent. There's nothing that distinctive about it. Some would say it's posh. Proper Essex and *EastEnders* would say it is, but real posh is the Queen (remember that lovely old lady who died?) and the cast of *Made in Chelsea* (who pronounce yeah as 'yah' and shorten Clapham Junction to 'Clappy J', basically Jamie Laing voice). My very mild Estuary twang doesn't have much of an accent to it unless a tradesperson comes into the house, in which case it's dialled right up so he thinks I'm a fackin' geezer. If you listen to old shows of mine on Radio 1, it's a lot more pronounced than it is now. I can't remember if that's how I was or whether I was putting it on a bit because I was on Radio 1. Probably a bit of both.

The posh thing always takes me by surprise because I don't see myself as fitting into any particular box, so being labelled in that way is an odd sensation. Maybe my surprise stems from not having a strong sense of cultural identity. I don't see myself as anything from anywhere, which isn't as bleak as I've made it sound. When people have a passionate connection to where they're from, it can be a really good shortcut to projecting who they are. I am often envious of people who can say, oh, I'm from Bolton or Birmingham or even Essex because you sort of 'get them' before you have a chance to get to know them. There are lots of areas in the UK with strong personalities and therefore, quite rightly, lots of people in the public eye will play on those roots. Sometimes it can be exhausting – we get it, you're from the north and you're dead normal and relatable despite being a multi-millionaire. I don't have that, however. Millions of people don't have that. You might be reading this now in suburbia thinking, *Yeah, Crawley's well boring!* (It is.) But look, this can be quite a good thing. There aren't any overriding preconceptions. No stereotyping. At school, I think I used not being from one fixed place to my advantage.

I hate it when people write boastfully about themselves as 'the outsider', thinking that it makes them more interesting. But because I moved so many times, I didn't ever fully get my feet under the table anywhere. So I was quite literally an outsider many times over, but I've always been quite happy floating around from group to group and being fairly unplaceable – and rather than ever really feeling like an outsider, I've always felt really in the middle. Maybe I was always like this or maybe my circumstances pointed me in this direction, but I've always loved observing people, noting their accents, their idiosyncrasies and then quite often learning to mimic them. I was part of the action at school – I certainly wasn't a loner – but I was also very rarely the ringleader. I really liked fitting in with different groups. Perhaps this goes back to the idea that in school, you're trying things out, working out who you are by process of elimination. In the summer, I'd be welcomed into the sporty crowd because I was really good at cricket, but aside from that, I loved being part of drama productions and helping to design the lighting and staging; I liked singing in the choir; I'd have a little group of friends who loved nerdy computer things, and another couple of mates who were into remote-controlled planes and we'd chat about air intakes and servos. When I got into the sixth form, I became a senior prefect (otherwise known as a senior brown-nose) and befriended a group of smart people who did clever things like running the school newspaper. They made me smarter as a result. I loved pushing myself even though they were top of the tree.

Who says you have to be one thing or have one group of friends and belong in one gang? I have always been lucky to get on with pretty much everyone. It's helped me immensely in my adult life. I can shapeshift! I can code switch! You don't know who I am from one minute to the next! And neither do I. But is that bad? Maybe. I don't know. I'm genuinely at my most comfortable in the middle of it all, able to adjust to whatever the situation needs. I find that fun. I always remember seeing my dad at work on the odd occasion when we all had to turn up to one of his school events and I'd be amazed at how he managed to interact with the kids one minute and then, at the drop of a hat, converse with a parent, a local politician or a governor. He was able to be all things to all people but you wouldn't immediately know where he was from and what his background was on first meeting. It's a good trick, I think. It's certainly useful for the radio. The joy of Radio 1 is that it's for people from all backgrounds and all ages to congregate together with the sole intention of having a nice time. Rich, poor, posh, smart, thick – whatever. And I love being one of the people that can help facilitate that. A bit like my dad used to do but in front of loads more people and for loads more money.

Imagine my surprise then, when I turned up at Radio 1 and was thrust into that incredible daytime line-up to do the *Early Breakfast Show* before Chris Moyles every day, only for him to start calling me a 'posh student'. I really wasn't expecting it. I mean, I don't help myself with the cricket thing. That can be an enormous posh red flag, or trouser, if you will. But it felt reductive to be called that. And it's something we're all guilty of. Moyles didn't know anything about me. He had no idea what my upbringing was like. He saw what he thought was a nice, excited, slightly boring 21-year-old student from the Home Counties with fantastic flowing indie hair who he could wind up a bit because I was new and just very happy to be there. And he was partly right. But I'd also managed to make my way to the best radio station in the world at a madly competitive time, so I was definitely up for the fight and eventually we had quite a funny on-air relationship where we'd take the piss out of each other. I guess I was just very bog-standard middle class and that wasn't interesting to him. And fair enough. I had to prove myself and also start working out who I was. So I'm actually grateful for the baptism of fire.

Showbiz lazily falls back on stereotypes a lot of the time, and panel-show bookings are often, *Oh, he's the geeky one, he'll be the deadpan one, she's the mean one and he'll be the thick twat.* I've never known where to fit into that world. I much prefer being the host, able to adopt lots of different personas depending on the situation. It's brilliant that people are more than one thing. We shouldn't be ashamed or confused about that. The idea of having several hats is a fundamental part of why I wanted to write this book in the first place. You're a different person at home from who you are at work, by and large. You speak differently to your mum than you do your best mates, or at least I hope you do, and you will behave differently in a group of strangers than in a pub full of mates you've known since you were 15. You'll find yourself being a slightly different version of yourself a lot over the course of even just one day. No matter where we're from, we are capable of shapeshifting many times over. Which is why it's important to fully work out who you are and which of the ways you present yourself is truly you before you make enormous life decisions. As well as this, we should all try as hard as possible to not judge someone too quickly just because we've spotted a particular calling card. Apart from wearing red trousers. They are almost certainly on the legs of a tosser.

I find class structures and where you're from and where you end up eternally fascinating. I grew up in the lower-middle class in a household where money was always a live issue. Luckily, not to the point of genuine hardship or destitution, but I was aware there wasn't much more than we needed. Which is of course fine, but it's the reason I still get stressed about it now. My parents will hate that I remember it but money chat was commonplace in the house and I got second-hand anxiety when debt or overdrafts were talked about. I'm definitely not tight with money but I'm very aware of how utterly horrible it is for it to be a worry that looms over you, so I've forced myself to be mindful of having a pension and all that boring stuff. Always being aware that there wasn't much money was a good lesson. At the risk of sounding like Keir Starmer here, wanging on about how his dad was a toolmaker, my mum, Rosemary, was from a lower-middle-class background and my dad, Alan, was from a working-class background and always lived in council houses. They both managed to get themselves into higher education and leave where they grew up to become teachers. My mum's dad was an estimator (someone who priced up how much construction things would cost) in the Midlands; her mum left school at 14 (!) and worked in a blanket factory nearby; my dad's mum worked in a grocer's in Witney; and his dad was a wool blender. So yeah, good solid jobs. My point is, they certainly weren't poshos or from money. We had a pretty modest house on Union Road in Bromley. I've just Google Street Viewed it. They've put new windows in since we were there and I don't like them. I was sad not to see a blue plaque saying, 'British Radio Legend Greg James (Milward) lived here … for a bit'. It's a nice suburban area with a decent little park around the corner (albeit a park that had a lot of dogshit in it in the 1990s, I seem to recall), a pub called the Chatterton Arms where my parents used to take me *a lot* and bribe me with lemonades and crisps in return for sitting there quietly for what felt like days, a newsagent's where I'd get my dad to buy me a couple of packs of Premier League stickers every Saturday, a bakery run by an old lady called Hilda who used to give me iced buns and a grocer's owned by a jolly man called Hasan who gave me a lot of cheese to try. In retrospect, my cheese obsession perhaps started here. Thank you, Hasan. It was good. A nice little community. Nothing special, but then I didn't know any different and I remember having a happy time there. Not everything has to be special or flashy or expensive. There's joy in the ordinary and I remember it all very fondly. Apart from Dog Shit Park.

All of this doesn't make me more interesting. It's just for information. In fact, it's very run of the mill. It's massively *unin-teresting*. Most people have lower-middle-class upbringings. What we were as a family, and I think my mum and dad would agree with this, was aspirational. We lived modestly but they were keen to give us a more financially comfortable life than they had. It tends to be like that in families. You want your kids to live a better life than you did. This was true of my mum and dad, who moved away from where they came from in search of a professional career. On teachers' salaries (which are disgustingly low), life was not luxurious but nor were we close to being on the streets. There was always food in the cupboards and a roast on the table on a Sunday. There was always a lot of music playing and time spent messing around in the garden and plenty of books around. It was a happy house. My parents were incredibly generous and worked themselves almost to death (in the case of my dad) to make sure my sister and I had a nice time. They stretched themselves so we could both go to university, have holidays, ride new bikes, get haircuts and wear nice trainers. That's what parents tend to do, isn't it? Their parents did it, my sister does it now for her kids and, well, I don't do that because I don't have any. But my dog, Barney, has such a great life. He doesn't realise how lucky he is. My sister and I felt loved, safe and happy. My mum and dad were and still are absolutely amazing and I'll never be able to repay them for what they've done for me.

I feel like I should probably expand on the 'dad nearly dying' thing I hinted at above. My dad is the most caring and considerate person I know. He is a very wise and funny man but a workaholic. He cared deeply about everyone who worked and studied at the school he was headmaster at in Enfield in the early to midnoughties, and that was his fatal flaw. Almost literally. He wore the stresses and strains and sadnesses of everyone, all of the time, to the point where he had to retire due to ill health at just 51. A mixture of a heart condition and mental burnout spelled the end for his teaching career and started an incredibly upsetting time for all of us but mostly Dad, who'd worked so hard to reach the dizzy heights of running a whole actual school. I'm grateful the plug was pulled when it was, though, because I wanted my dad around more than I wanted him to be a headteacher. No job is worth that. This all happened when I was in my mid-teens, deep in school exams and trying to work out who I was. It certainly made me grow up quickly and it was a very abrupt reminder that life is short, adults are fallible and nothing is ever certain. My dad descended into a pretty dark depression because he couldn't square that he was no longer doing the job he loved and that he wasn't providing for the family. It's understandable if that's the mark of success you've made for yourself but a great lesson to me to make sure your self-worth isn't too tied up in your career. There was also the very real panic of a loss of quite a big chunk of income, meaning that my mum had to keep working longer than she would have probably liked, so my dad felt guilty about that too. But, as a family, we huddled around him and did our very best to remind him of why we loved him. It certainly wasn't for his stupid job that kept him out of the house all day and most of the evening. I now had my dad back. But for a while, he was a shell of himself. It was extremely tough for all of us but you have to keep going and I'm so pleased to say that despite the odd appearance from the Black Dog (depression, not Barney), he is happy, well and fully nestled into his OAP lifestyle. But it's been a process – one that made the family stronger and my bond with my old man unbreakable. I feel weirdly lucky that I had to go through that relatively young because it meant that I stepped up to help my parents, was there for them and perhaps shut down excessive teenage selfishness because there were more important things going on.

This perspective has no doubt impacted how I approach my day-to-day life. Growing up around someone with a mental illness serves as an early reminder that life is complicated (as is your brain) and sometimes frightening. Dad's dark times have given me a huge dollop of perspective and provided me with a healthy grounding when the petty woes of my job or frivolous celebrity nonsense threaten my peace. I'm careful to try to not let my job interfere with my real life too often. Dad is living proof that you can give too much. That you can care too much. I don't want to go to that place. His troubles also serve as a constant reminder to be aware of what others might be going through privately. Mum and Dad are empaths and I'm lucky to have inherited that from them. It serves me incredibly well in my job as it means I'm always curious when talking to someone new. I love finding out what makes people tick. In fact I like finding out what makes *me* tick! Even if those things are uncomfortable.

I spoke to my friend Matt about this chapter (for *Tailenders* listeners, that's Mattchin) and he remarked on how much he loves seeing me and my dad out and about at cricket together. I love involving my parents in the fun things I get invited to and I value my friendships with them so much. I can never fully repay them for the life they gave me but the odd trip to the hospitality suite at Lords, a look at the nice flowers at Hampton Court or hanging out with the poshos at Wimbledon goes some of the way. One of the best times was when I took my mum to watch the tennis and we were in the same box as James Norton, who she has an enormous crush on. She kept complimenting him on his 'lovely pink suit'. Get a grip, Rosemary.

I feel like I should admit that in my quieter, more reflective moments, I think that having children of my own might be worth it just to have the relationship with them that I enjoy with my parents now. But that's not enough of a reason. There's a lot to get through and sacrifice before you get into a position where this friendship might happen. And *might* is the crucial word. It's a gamble. That sort of bond is rare and just because I'm experiencing it with my parents doesn't mean it would definitely happen if I had kids. You have to get lucky that your parents turn into great friends, and I feel like I won the double rollover on that one so that's enough for me. I already *am* part of this friendship dynamic. I don't need to try to recreate it with me in the parental role.

The sadness my dad felt at this time was largely due to the fact that he thought he'd failed in some way. His narrative from when he was a young man was *work hard, push yourself, make a good life for yourself and your family* – and suddenly this plan had stalled. He felt an invisible pressure, perhaps from society and his upbringing, that if he didn't have the big job and couldn't elevate himself through the class system, he was worthless. It's a dangerous track to find yourself on, putting all your self-worth on a career. But we are obsessed with class and wealth and social mobility.

The obsession is uniquely British. It's not particularly healthy but it gives us all something to talk about and I get sucked into it, too. For example, I'm deeply judgemental when I see a new plummy-voiced actor spring onto the scene and I'm straight onto Wikipedia to find out which very expensive boarding school he went to. Again, reducing everyone to one thing is lazy and dangerous, but we *all* do it. One of the traps is that it's too straightforward to say that everyone in the upper class or 'posh' is rich. Similarly, it's wrong to say all working-class people are poor. This intersection of class vs. wealth played out beautifully on the David Beckham documentary on Netflix from a couple of years ago. Victoria Beckham has literally been known for 30 years as 'Posh Spice'. She was born in a town next to Bishop's Stortford called Harlow. Anyone that knows Harlow will know that it is not in the least bit posh. Her dad, Tony, started a very successful electrical wholesale business and apparently made a lot of money in the 1980s, giving the family a very comfortable life. David called her out on her claim that she was 'working class' in the documentary because her dad drove a Rolls-Royce. This is a *classic* British confusion where he's equating money to class. Her mum was a hairdresser and her dad was an electrical engineer. That isn't exactly landed gentry, is it? Neither are they what you'd call traditional 'white collar' or 'professional' jobs like lawyers, doctors, etc. They are a working family who did very well for themselves. This is where it's complicated. But the fact is, actual proper posh people who have estates and family money from hundreds of years ago and go shooting and eat pheasant (no offence, Victoria) would think she was as common as muck (again, no offence, Victoria). No matter how much money you earn, you'll never be able to make it into the upper class. You're born into it. Just watch *Saltburn* to work it all out.

Depending on your upbringing, you'll have your own analysis of what I am. And of course what everyone else is. It's all about perspective. I joke that I'm Bella's bit of rough. Compared to her upper-middle-class north London childhood, mine is much more reminiscent of Oliver Twist's. I was astounded to see how her family lived. For the first time, I saw signifiers of wealth and class that I hadn't before. Moth-ridden cushions and blankets, shabby/scruffy decor, mismatched patterns, old crockery from Granny, an open fireplace, worn carpets and a disregard for keeping your car clean are all dead giveaways of a fairly well-to-do family. Slightly down the rung, achingly middle-class families like mine tend to keep things clean and tidy, have dinner plates they keep 'for best', mow the grass regularly, have a shoes-off policy on the new carpets and take great pride in a clean car. It's mad that we can build up a picture of an entire family by what food they had in the house. Bella once told me that when she was a child, Italian amaretti biscuits would be passed around the table after dinner. She said, as if it was something ALL children did, that the biscuits came in a nice wrapper that they'd then light, which turned them into lanterns that would float serenely around the dining room. I just told Bella I'm writing this bit and she's watching over me. I'm telling her what sort of desserts would be on offer after Sunday lunch in the 1990s in my house. Treacle tart, lemon meringue pie or crumble and custard, usually. 'Homemade?' she asked. I just burst out laughing. They were always shop-bought. Thanks to *Bake Off*, things might be different now, and perhaps I'd serve up a biscuit in the shape of Clare Balding's face (this is what I made when I was on that show) but back then essentially the options were maybe a mint Viennetta, or perhaps Sara Lee would lend a hand. How the other half live, eh? Oh, and cleaners. Ironically, Bella's parents' house looks like it's never been cleaned and yet someone comes in once a week to push the dust around and entertain the moths a bit.

My mum and dad would be horrified if anyone was employed to clean their house. I recommended that Mum got a cleaner once, and she not only cleaned before she came round but had to leave the house when she did. And when she returned home, she'd go over what she'd done. Sadly, the cleaner didn't last long. My mum didn't kill her, she just said she didn't want her to come anymore. As I write this, I'm sitting in a house that was decorated by Bella, on a shabby old sofa, in a room covered in floral granny wallpaper realising just how far I've come. I've infiltrated those higher echelons, guys! I've made it! Moth kingdom! Well, actually, I haven't. You can't change. That's the horror and simultaneous beauty of these systems and strata that humans have invented. No amount of money will ever make me truly posh. And I'm fine with that. I have to be. That said, I'd love to have had very rich grandparents leave me a manor house or something. I'd fully Barry Keoghan it in the drawing room every single day. Curtains open, Ellis-Bextor on the speakers, cock fully out.

It's ludicrous to think of my life now compared to what it used to be like. I'm still the same person with the same values but I now live in a place I never even realised existed. It wasn't accessible to me before I got successful. Central-ish London. It's the biggest house I've ever lived in. And it's mine. ALL MINE. Well, with a quite a big mortgage, but I bought it with the money I made, not money I got given from a rich parent, annoyingly. That would have been much easier. But I'm proud of that. The contrast between what my grandparents had and what I have now is ridiculous. And there isn't a day that goes by where I don't feel simultaneously amazed by that and also incredibly lucky.

All the best for the future

Maybe that's why, despite me saying it doesn't matter what your background is, it riles me a bit when people call me posh, because none of this was ever handed to me. I'm still Greggy from the Block (well, Union Road), no more or less happy than I was with not as much money – that's famously not the way things correlate. Who's to say I wouldn't find just as much joy from carrying on the family tradition of teaching? Oh, and yes, I have a cleaner now. I hate myself a bit. But I *love* how Ana makes our bed. She does the hotel tuck on the duvet. It's incredible. Also, she and Barney are an amazing double act. He lies around doing farts as she vacuums around him.

Give Us
a Job,
Mate?

If you were lucky enough to grow up in a relatively safe, nourishing environment it probably felt like anything was possible for your future when you were a kid. Imagining what you could do probably started with the big famous jobs like footballer, astronaut (if you're Katy Perry) or spy. You're told that all these things are achievable so your hopes get dashed when you get a bit older and you see that for most people, jobs involve putting on weirdly formal clothes you'd never normally wear, commuting on a hot, smelly train and sitting in an office desperately waiting for 5pm to tick round. It's bizarre that when you pick your GCSEs, you're barely a teenager and yet you're starting to steer yourself towards a career. No way is that healthy. Oh, sorry, I thought we were irresponsible hormone-fuelled idiots? It was only a couple of years ago that you told us that we could become dinosaur hunters or princesses and now you're saying we might need to plan for the eventuality that the reality might be less Jurassic Park and more drinks at BOXPARK after another classic day moving money around for J.P. Morgan? Suddenly we're making decisions that might affect the rest of our lives, are we? MAKE UP YOUR MINDS!

How are you supposed to know what you want to do at that age? This stuff isn't easy and there are many potential jobs to do: good ones, bad ones, easy ones, hard ones, shit ones, evil ones, boring ones, fun ones, famous ones, pointless ones. It's a mine-field. (There are jobs on those too. 'Dangerous jobs' is another category I should add.) But whatever type of job you have, and yours *will* fall into one of my very well-thought-through categories above, it shouldn't define you. And yet we've made a society where it does. It can feel like you're choosing a fixed personality when you figure out what career is for you. In between astronaut and accountant are a million other paths people can take to 'make a living'. I ask people what they do for a living all the time, multiple times a day in fact on the radio when I'm talking to callers. It's a quick way to get a memorable fact from someone but it's also quite reductive. I'll have a fantastic caller on the *Breakfast Show* who's got a life populated with people they love, things they're passionate about, dreams they want to fulfil, places they want to visit, and there I am reducing their entire personality down to the simple fact of what they get up early for to make cash. You some-times get interesting answers like Ellie, who once called up to do a funny bit on the show and before we got to the feature she replied to my job question by saying that she was in charge of putting the coffins on the conveyor belt at a crematorium in Norfolk. I mean, that's absolute gold. And a job I can't imagine she had in mind when she was choosing her GCSE options. I can't even remember why she called up, so I'm not saying it's a *bad* question, but maybe it shouldn't be the first or only one.

They say, 'Do something you love and you'll never work a day in your life,' but do you have to do a job you love? I've always worried about this phrase. It feels like it might have been invented by a monstrous CEO to keep productivity and 'vibes' high. That very intense, bald Scottish bloke from BrewDog went viral for this recently, didn't he? The implication being, 'Work is so fun, you don't need other fun because work gives you all the fun!' Let's be under no illusions here: most people are working for nothing more than a salary. This isn't to say that work *can't* be enjoyable, but thinking it *has* to be can take you down a dangerous path.

I'd take a stab that most people don't do jobs they love, or even like. I'm one of the smug pricks that somehow ended up doing the job I wanted to do when I was a teenager and I love it as much as I hoped I would then, if not more. But I don't know if the love I have for my job is that healthy. Who's to say I'm happier than someone who does a day's work, packs up, leaves it all in the office and doesn't think about it again until the next day they turn up? Again, you are not your job. It can be a fabulous, enriching, wonderful part of your life but it really shouldn't define you because if it goes, then what happens to you? I refer you back to my dad. A job shouldn't be a substitution for the truly important things in life. A job can *feel* like it's giving you that, but ultimately, it's transactional. A ruthless boss. A (possibly evil) company that doesn't care about you. It wants you to give all of yourself over to it, and it'll take as much as you give and then ask for more. Before you know it, working late becomes the norm to try to get on top of all the work you want to do to 'impress' and to 'get on', but you'll never be 'done' with this attitude. The workload will keep growing because they think you can manage it, the amount of time you have in a day never increases and you'll end up burnt out like a husk. Sometimes it's good to treat your job and its management structure with the disdain with which it treats you. I'll think of some more interesting ice-breaker questions for the callers on my show. Maybe 'Do you prefer dogs or cats?', 'Name a famous person with the same first name as you' or 'When did you last have a McFlurry?' My answers, by the way: dogs (obviously), Greg Davies and on the way back from Radio 1's Big Weekend in Liverpool this year. A McFlurry is a top-tier mid-five-hour-journey energy boost.

Although being a radio presenter is a dream job, it's not the *only* dream I've ever had. It won't surprise you to learn that being a 'Chuckle Brother' was definitely an ambition at one point. One of the many reasons this could never have happened is I can't grow a moustache, plus I wasn't born into the Chuckle Dynasty. I was also very keen on being a firefighter, mainly because of *Fireman Sam* and an obsession with fire engines. This is an obsession I still have. Bella laughs at me every time I see one because I'll stop mid-sentence to enjoy it thundering past, sirens hooting and howling, lights blinking manically. Cumbersome yet majestic. I've been laughed at by friends because I often look at the second-hand fire engine market and when I excitedly tell them you can get a good Dennis appliance (that's what us pros call fire engines) for about £5,000 if you wanted, they look at me as if I've just loudly shat myself. Oh my god, I'd love to drive around in an old fire engine. It's such a statement, such a vibe. It would give me a new edge and make me immediately more interesting. Maybe *that's* the 'thing' I need! 'Oh yeah, did you hear that Greg James has a 1990s fire engine as his daily drive?' In the spirit of this book and encouraging everyone to do things the ten-year-old them would love, maybe I should buy a cheap fire engine which everyone can use if they want. Hire it out for weddings or whatever. I also spent quite a long time imagining a life as a bus driver. Maybe I just love the idea of driving big old wagons. On walks with my mum and dad as a kid I remember zooming ahead on the path pretending to be a double-decker and making the hissing noises a bus does when it stops to pick people up.

As well as spending several hours fantasising about driving things, I also thought I might be a professional cricketer, a stunt man, a special effects coordinator, a TV camera operator and at one point, James Bond. But not an actor that gets the role of James Bond, an actual spy who works for MI6 with the exact same exciting, glamorous life that James Bond leads but with a stipulation that I would never die. That would be a deal breaker. I was so obsessed with the idea of being James Bond that I once took my first girlfriend up to London to visit the exterior of the secret Tube station door on Westminster Bridge which featured in the (Pierce Brosnan, my hero, aside) dreadful 2002 Bond film, *Die Another Day*. She didn't share my excitement as I skipped up the steps shouting, 'That's it! That's it! The Bond door!' Like lots of toxic men, I firmly believe I would be a brilliant spy. I love driving nice cars, hanging out with nice moody women and hiding from people, I'm vain about my appearance and I truly, truly hate bad guys. Why hasn't the Ministry of Defence got in touch? I have genuinely thought this through and I often wonder whether it crossed their minds to ask me to be a spy but then they thought, *Oh, hang on, he can't do that because he's a minor national treasure.* I've had the counterargument in my head for a while just in case. I'd challenge this reasoning by saying that I'm in fact the perfect candidate to be a spy.

No one would ever suspect the silly man off the radio of also being a trained killer, would they? Look at it this way: it's the perfect cover. I might be a spy and you'll never know! This whole book could be part of the deception and I've been hiding in plain sight all this time. The baddies would never suspect me, would they? Come to think of it, the actors that have played James Bond would be the perfect people to go and do a bit of freelance espionage for the government. Send Daniel Craig to go and keep an eye on Putin! Get hold of Brosnan and arrange a meet and greet with Xi Jinping! But make sure he takes photos and gets up close and personal with his wife or whatever to get information. Lazenby and Dalton to a lesser extent, though. They might well be working for the government and no one would ever know. To be honest, they could have MOT'd your car last week and you wouldn't have realised. Apart from maybe noticing the seats were fully reclined when you picked it up. Some things never change.

What else do I genuinely think I could do? I realise that this is the most Alan Partridge chapter of the book so far but I could be a pilot. Definitely. Commercial, though. I'm a lover not a fighter. I went and hung out with the Red Arrows earlier this year and I don't think I could manage the formation stuff or the precision loop-de-loops either. None of the Ryanairs I've been on so far have done any of that stuff so I reckon with a few goes in the simulator, I'd be able to give that a go. Maybe they could ease me in by being the first officer just so I can get the hang of it and nail the radio stuff. That's where I'd shine. I'd be absolutely amazing on the PA doing a version of the *Breakfast Show*, playing a few tunes, telling people what Timothée Chalamet's been up to and endlessly repeating funny animal clips. If we ever got held on the runway while waiting for a take-off slot I could do a round of Unpopular Opinion with the passengers. 'I hate having to listen to the boring safety announcement!' would be mine. 'They say all planes are slightly different, but they're really not *that* different. And to be honest, in the event of an emergency, no one's going to take kindly to the nerd blocking the inflatable slide saying, 'Well if you'd *listened* earlier, you'd know that you don't need to take your shoes off on an Airbus slide, that's only for the 737's ...' 'Oh, SHUT UP!' I'd yell as I pushed him out the door and into the North Sea.

I also think I'd be a brilliant ghost. I don't really believe in ghosts but I'm very up for the idea. I've just never seen one and I wish I had some proof to go off. I'd love to be as sure about ghosts as some people are (normally Facebook aunties, let's be honest). I know it's a devastating thought but at some point I will die. Sorry to break it to you, but hopefully it won't be for ages – I often think how annoyed I'd be if it all came to an end now. I would be completely furious. The fury would be lessened, however, if I'd be allowed back as a ghost. If this happened, I would be such a nuisance. First port of call would be the Global Radio building, mainly so I could go and shit up Amanda Holden a bit. Re-edit some of the songs to include swear words, let her chair down while she's mid-sentence, keep turning the lights on and off, put some rude place names in the travel news – that sort of fare. Nothing too mean. I'd go and pull Chris Moyles's trousers down and re-patch the Capital broadcast feed so it played out a livestream of PornHub. I'd maybe even go and visit Alan Sugar and ride up and down on his Stannah stairlift in the middle of the night. Maybe also fill up his walk-in bath and populate it with rubber ducks that have his head.

Anyway, where was I? Is there a point to any of this? Yes! We can get so focused on *what* we want to be when we grow up that we forget that it's more important (and more fun) to work out *who* we want to be. I get that it's easy to use your job as a useful shorthand for telling people a bit about yourself but let's make sure we're not all work and no play. At the end of your life, is it more important for you to be thought of as a really brilliant, supportive partner and friend or an expert coder? The most generous and kind brother or the person who whipped up the best spreadsheets for the quarterly sales review? You can be all of these things of course, but what's more important to you?

Did I Mention I Love Radio?

I still wake up every day and have a moment where I can't quite believe I managed to get onto Radio 1. That feeling spurs me on every morning and when I feel tired or out of ideas it jolts me into action. The day I got 'the call' lives so vividly in my head, I can remember everything about it. I was on holiday with my mum, dad and my girlfriend Clare. I was 21 and had just graduated from university. We were all in the garden of the place we were staying in the South of France as my phone rang and I rushed inside to answer it. I was looking out over them from a balcony above listening intently as my agent, Chris North, recounted a meeting he'd just had with the then Head of Programmes, Ben Cooper, where he'd offered me the *Early Breakfast Show* full-time, five days a week starting in October. Just a few months earlier, I'd almost been tempted to accept another job offer at Galaxy Radio in Birmingham, and, although I'd been very excited about it, I'd wanted to hold out for the big one. And thank fuck I did. The Galaxy gig would have been an incredible first step into the radio industry, and I'd been happy with the offer of £18k a year for it. So it blew my mind that Ben Cooper was about to put me on the most famous radio station in the world and pay me £80k a year. I cried. Immediately. I hung up, ran outside to my family and said, 'It's happened.' The thing I quietly always thought could happen if I was lucky, DID happen.

After a huge hug and a dance around, I decided to grab the keys to the hire car (a Toyota Yaris) and drove myself around the rugged French hills,* screaming along to 'Apply Some Pressure' by Maxïmo Park on repeat. I remember Clare checking to see if I was OK because of my insistence that it be a solo drive. At the time, I couldn't explain why I wanted to do this but in hindsight it's because doing radio was a little secret quest I'd set out on alone all those years previously. It felt right just to take myself off and sit in that moment to try to come to terms with it. It was the happiest I'd ever felt – a childhood dream realised and I couldn't believe it. I still can't. Lots of brilliant people helped me achieve that first job, my parents and Clare included, but just for a brief moment, I wanted to try to make sense of things.

My first ever live show on Radio 1 was only a couple of months before I got that call on 1 June 2007. It was a very warm morning. I remember this because it followed a very hot and uncomfortable night in the Holiday Inn around the corner. I didn't sleep at all. Of course I didn't. Only maniacs would get a relaxing night's sleep before being unleashed on national radio for the first time. I was practising my first link over and over while staring at the ceiling until finally it was time to get up. I switched the wall-mounted TV on and played Radio 1 as I was having a shower and couldn't believe that in under two hours, I'd be the one making the songs come out of those speakers – and, of course, speakers all over the country. I now make a point of cycling past that Holiday Inn on the way home every day after the *Breakfast Show* because it reminds

---

* I don't recall a boner this time.

me of the terror and excitement of that morning. On this day in 2007, however, I was walking towards the studio on an unusually quiet Great Portland Street. There were very few cars on the road and only the odd person stumbling home after a big Thursday night as the beginnings of a new day were being pieced together. A bin lorry wheezed its way down the street, a few birds had their say on proceedings, and there was that warm, hazy stillness that indicates a hot and sticky summer's day was on the cards. The mundane, functional serenity of a city waking up was just what I needed to help root myself in reality before going to do something absolutely mad.

I loved every second of the show. I made the most of it. I tried to take it all in and enjoy it all. It was, of course, overwhelming. But I enjoyed being overwhelmed. It was entirely appropriate to feel like that. And in any case, I was in safe hands. A great man called Neil Sloan was my producer. He had championed me from my student radio days and is instrumental in completely changing my life. He'll be embarrassed to be mentioned in the book but, love you, Neilos. We did it! We did the *Early Breakfast Show* for two years and they're still some of my favourite shows I've ever done.

Without doubt the highlight of that first morning came at ten past five when Dave Vitty (Comedy Dave) from *The Chris Moyles Show* poked his head around the door and said, 'Sounding great this morning.' Coming from him, a man I'd listened to for years at school, this meant so much. Even if it wasn't true, he clearly knew how much I loved being there, he could hear how hard I was trying and how excited I was to be there and it did the trick. I immediately felt at home and more relaxed. I learnt from that.

Whenever there's a new person on now and I pass their studio, I remember what Dave did and I do the same to them if they're showing some promise and trying their best. If they're really shit, however, I'll just walk past quickly, pretend to be late and wave.

The other vivid memory I revisit often is of launching *The Radio 1 Breakfast Show* in 2018. This was the day the dream turned into something I could never really have imagined. I was 33 when I took over that show and, as I said in my opening link, in a weird way I'd been preparing for that first show for 20 years. It was not only full of bits that my team and I had lovingly prepared and planned in the weeks leading up to the launch, but beneath the surface it contained all the years of work – and play – that had led me to that point. I'd done all my existential overthinking in the days leading up to it, but five minutes before pressing play on that opening theme tune, I was unbelievably calm. It surprised me. But it's because I knew exactly what I was doing and knew precisely what I wanted to say to everyone. 'Hello, I'm Greg and I love radio so much.' That was my truth and it still is. I was simultaneously the 12-year-old me and the 33-year-old me and it's a morning I'll never forget. I was part of the most brilliant team for that launch, headed up by Will Foster and Chris Sawyer, the two most talented creative brains that have ever set foot in Radio 1. We had a clear mission statement: make it funny, make it silly, play great songs and, most importantly, make it all about the listeners. Trust them, make them part of the fun, make them the stars, get to know them, celebrate them and be there for them. Create as big a gang of wonderful weirdos as possible. And my role was simple. I was to be the Ringleader, the conductor of this mad orchestra of nonsense ideas. I remember thinking, *I can absolutely do this.* Those rushes of confidence and clarity are rare and I'm so lucky to have been in a position to experience that. I felt totally in control and giddy with happiness and that three-hour show changed my life; because it was deemed a success, I've been able to keep on doing it ever since. I'm so proud it's still going. If I never experience a high like that again in my professional life, it won't matter because I had that one. And it was the best one.

The deal you make when you agree to do a show like this is that you will turn up every day, no matter how you feel, and do your best to spread some joy and have fun. It won't always be exciting and exhilarating. You won't always feel happy, for one thing – no one is – and that's when you have to really prove you love it. I'm fortunate that my general disposition is an optimistic one, but even the most annoyingly chirpy characters were tested in March 2020 when Covid took hold and the country was locked down.

As an aside, before I force you to think back to that time, do you remember how much we used to take the piss out of people who called it 'Covid'? You'd have been called a fucking square for that in 2020. In fact, I remember Michael Gove referring to it as 'COV-ID' and everyone laughing at him because he said the 'co' like you do when you say 'Coventry' and not like when you say 'coach'. He also said that a Scotch egg was a substantial meal while we were all panicking about what we could eat and where and with whom, so maybe we can't trust anything he says. But yes, we all used to call it coronavirus and now it's Covid.

But whatever you call it, it was a complete nightmare and changed the world, and probably all of us, forever. All in all, it was a bleak time. Now I'm not a complete monster and don't think for one second that what we did on the radio was in any way comparable to the genuine sacrifices that others made, but reframing *The Radio 1 Breakfast Show* and constantly shifting and reacting to what was happening in the world was the most challenging thing I've ever done.

I'd never considered that I might be broadcasting to millions of worried people. Tired people? Sure! Terrified? Lost? Sad? Grief-stricken? Poorly? Yes, a few, but not on the scale we saw. I was all of these things myself over the course of those couple of years. Which helped, I guess. I needed to do that show just as much as people needed us to do it, needed to hear something familiar and reassuring. It's calming to have the relative normality of the voices you know still floating over the airwaves. Radio has always served as an extraordinary lifeline and connection, or, when it's needed, a disconnection from whatever the outside world throws at us. And on this occasion the world threw us a huge ball of shit. But it was nothing we couldn't deal with and it was a pleasure to be tasked with making sure our listeners were looked after and heard.

The 'YOU MUST STAY AT HOME' narrative was deliberately loud and clear from the government but us lot on the radio were all too aware of the reality of our listeners' lives. Most people CAN'T stay at home and do their job. Yeah sure, fantastic if you've got a job that you could do from anywhere, but if you're delivering things, mending stuff or working in healthcare or education, it's not quite as easy. We were there for those who *had* to go out and brave it. And by brave it, I mean risk their lives. We should have been banging our pots and pans for the truckers every Thursday as well as NHS staff, come to think of it. But that really was what we were aiming to do on the *Breakfast Show* every day: be there for the listeners, provide a distraction and celebrate those who were still going out there and doing their bit. My 'bit' was relatively safe and I do feel uncomfortable when people say to me 'thanks for being there in those dark days' because the listeners got me through too, so I'm the one who should be grateful. The bond between me, the listeners and radio as an entity was strengthened over the course of those two years.

I truly understood radio's meaning and power, and doing that show was not only the ultimate test as a presenter but also an enormous privilege. The way the team navigated those treacherous waters while also finding time to splosh around and have fun is the thing I'll be most proud of when my time at Radio 1 comes to an end, whenever that may be. Doing a whole campaign to get a person from every country in the world to shout 'UP YOURS, CORONA' and reworking Alphabeat's 'Fascination' to 'VACCI-NATION!' on the morning the Pfizer vaccine was rolled out will always make me look back with pride at how we dealt with it. 'Can you do this show when everything's gone to shit, please?' The answer was 'Yes, just about.'

Holy
Shit

The weeks leading up to Christmas are my favourite time of the year. Even if you're working, it tends to be a quiet period, unless you're a medical professional, or Father Christmas. In general, most people get a bit of time off, the work emails slow down to a standstill and the days start merging into one. The Christmas period is one of my top basic things that I love. Along with New York and pizza. I'm a basic bitch. I love the decorations that brighten up the dark, dreary days, I love having a licence to use Baileys as a milk substitute in coffee and opening a calendar that gives you a chocolate every morning. I love putting a tree up in my house. I love getting to play Christmas songs on the radio as I get to share everyone else's excitement at some pending time off. I love 'Christmas pub' with its cheap shiny decorations and steamed-up windows, with everyone in a great mood, more pissed than usual. I love the rush of finishing things off or catching up with people 'before Christmas' like it's the end of the world even though it's only days. Soon enough and we'll all be back to normal, after the turkey carcass has been boiled down and only the pathetic Bountys are left stranded in the Celebrations tub. The period between Christmas and New Year's Day is the most immovable thing in everyone's diary. A full stop on the year. This natural conclusion to the year forces you to look back and assess your own progress as a human. Your very own slightly drunken end-of-year review. It can be useful but it can also be harrowing if you've had a bad year. But therein lies one of the problems with it. Why do we all measure life in year-long strands?

Why does a year have to be either good or bad? The year, if you want to count it as one important passage of time, is full of all sorts of days. Good ones, bad ones, boring ones, bleak ones, happy ones, sad ones, memorable ones, forgettable ones. It's a very emotionally charged time of year and we're all forced to look back and reflect; it brings our lives into sharp focus. And for many, that's not a particularly healthy exercise.

I've always considered December 25th itself the most over-rated day of all. Perhaps I'm being contrary in an attempt to be interesting but I've always hated big days that everyone's forced to get excited about. Valentine's Day is one of the worst offenders: it's so naff. Mother's Day and Father's Day are lame and just serve to make my friends who've lost a parent really sad. There's too much pressure to have fun on New Year's Eve and the weather's always shit, and don't get me started on April Fool's Day. It's the ultimate in forced fun and is only really for people who don't get to be fun every day. For those of us that are lucky enough to be able to piss around every day, April Fool's Day is actually a welcome day off where I'll put on a suit and tie, stick on Radio 3 and spend the day seeing how the economy is doing.

The main problem with Christmas Day is that there's too much riding on it. It's over-planned, overthought and overhyped. A bit like the Brit Awards. We've had such a nice build-up with all the festivities I mentioned above that we feel it needs to culminate somewhere, so we all get carried away and then, when the day arrives, how can it possibly give us the pay-off we need? We expect too much from it. Christmas is a great example of the journey being better than the destination. And I forget this every year. I feel ridiculous if I'm sad on Christmas Day. But why should I? I don't feel bad for feeling like shit on the 16th of May. So why do I feel like I've let myself, my family and the entire year down if I have a bad December 25th? There's a pressure to savour every moment of the day. To create meaningful memories, cook the best food, ensure everyone's having a nice time, all get along, not put a finger out of place as if we're all going to be marked by the Christmas Ofsted inspectors at the end of it. Here's a bold suggestion: maybe scatter a few of the things we try to cram into Christmas Day throughout the year. Catch up with those family members at a different, less intense juncture, maybe? Have more regular, less pressurised gatherings with your friends and family when you're not knackered, skint and stressed, perhaps?! I try to do this but I still fall into the same traps. As I sit down to Christmas dinner, there's a voice telling me this has to be the very best meal of the year. You must be engaging, funny, interested. Your very best, happiest self. This *must* go down as a classic dinner. We're all putting on such a weird show. Performative joy.

I have always worried about someone close to me dying around Christmas. Obviously because it would be incredibly upsetting, but also because for the rest of your life, you'll have to traverse a time of year where we've made sure there's only room for celebration and joy. Sorry, mate, is there any way your nan could hold on a couple of weeks so we can push your sadness into January, please? I'm trying to wrap bacon around a sausage while wearing a paper hat.

In my early teens, when the greedy excitement of the presents bit of it wore off, I became aware of the upheaval of it all. The money and energy the whole thing requires. Christ! Literally. I don't know how my mum and dad didn't just sit around crying all of Christmas Day. Perhaps they wanted to. Perhaps they did. But you're not allowed to show any chink in the armour, are you? Don't wince. Everyone *must* act like they're having a nice time. Even if they're not. The brave-facing of it from all parties is a collective madness, but the pressure and stress parents are under at that time of year makes me despair. A counter-argument to this slight rant I'm enjoying is that Christmas is for the kids. And yes, I do see that. I loved the excitement of Father Christmas appearing magically in the night and leaving an old sock on my bed. But are we doing kids a disservice by pushing Christmas Day too hard? I grew up with the unrealistic notion that Christmas Day had to be perfect and flawless. And if it wasn't, it was a failure. Maybe we need to reappraise it. What do we actually want to do on Christmas Day? Be honest with ourselves. Do we want to see the people we see or do we feel obliged? Maybe it is time for us all to pare it back a bit. Especially if you're not a Christian. It's supposed to be a celebration of Jesus. He'd be horrified if he saw us devouring a week's worth of food in two hours and then just doing farts for the rest of the day.

Shall we talk about the true meaning of Christmas? Don't worry, I'm not going to be one of those exhausting people that bangs on about being an atheist. Why do you care so much? Let people have a nice thing that's important to them. In my early twenties I was much punchier about rubbishing religion. It was fun to trick myself into thinking I was so sure about something. It felt like I'd cracked the code and everyone else with their little Bibles and church services was stupid. But with age, you learn to appreciate and understand other people and their beliefs and views. And when you dig into why, you should be left with no doubt that what people choose to believe in should be respected. Even if it sounds completely fucking batshit.

Togetherness is what everyone craves. To feel less alone in the world. And it's a tough world to traverse, so why wouldn't you want to try to make sense of some of it by believing in a god? Or many. One isn't nearly enough if you're Hindu. They're having a laugh, aren't they? It's a lovely thing and something I wish I believed. I'm jealous of people who feel that pull. The sense of community, a shared belief system geared towards helping each other, is really wonderful. The idea of being part of something bigger is appealing but I just can't get on board because of, well, for me, science. I suppose I'm an agnostic. You can't prove it one way or the other so the sensible thing to say is, 'I don't know.' A bit like 'Does my dog understand what I'm saying to him?' Probably not, but I'll never truly know.

Christmas Day itself would have a much clearer objective if I was a Christian, though, and I do really love a good carol service. As long as it's the well-known ones. I went to one last Christmas and they didn't play any of the hits so I walked out mid-song. My editor has asked me to add in the carols I was expecting. Charlotte, come on! The readers know a Christmas banger! They don't need to be told *everything*. But for the record, I was expecting your 'Once in Royal David's City's, your 'Oh! Come All Ye Faithful's, your 'Hark the Herald Angels Sing', 'Silent Night', 'O Little Town of Bethlehem.' ... You know! The big ones. Anyway, I got out of there after the third obscure deep-cut started. That's called knowing yourself.

You know what *is* a good day, though? The best day of the year? Christmas Eve. Now we're talking. Sure, tomorrow we'll have an intense and emotionally exhausting day of acting like everything's fine even if it's not, so today ... let's forget all our troubles and cut loose. Christmas Eve pub is the best pub. If you find the right one — sweaty and small, ideally — then you can feel like you're on the bottom deck of the *Titanic*. You know the bit of the film — with Jack and Rose doing Irish dancing. Rose pretending she likes the dirty working-class people down there? Stick The Pogues on and you've got yourself a 10/10 night where anything goes. That's what Christmas Eve should feel like if you get it right. It's particularly great if you're single and something happens. Everyone's much more up for it at Christmas. Maybe it's the cold. (It's not, it's the alcohol.)

Advice from a Smug Prick

Along with how we let Logan and Jake Paul become famous and why so many people still watch *The Apprentice*, LOVE will always be one of life's biggest mysteries. And that's how it's supposed to be, annoyingly. Being in love is at times absolutely hideous. When it's going right, it's without question the most blissful feeling a human can experience. But this is life, remember! And the flip side of that dizzy high is the devastating low if it all goes tits up. Love is wonderful, until it's not, and it can turn horrible quickly. You have to be prepared for every emotion; all the colours will be on display, especially the dark ones. When you fall in love, you make a deal to open yourself up to the potential of the greatest joy imaginable but the gamble is that you're left wide open to immense pain. The whole world is obsessed with it. Most songs, most stories, most films and most art is about love. Or just as often, a sudden lack of it. It's a big topic but I think I'm the man to tackle it. Hey, I've just celebrated my seventh wedding anniversary so I think I know a thing or two.

I've been at my happiest when I've been in love but also my absolute rock-bottom lowest. Love can be devious and you only need to take a look at the source material to realise this. I've always distrusted Cupid, for example. He's a smug prick, isn't he? Just hovering around shooting people with arrows. You'd be arrested for doing that on Oxford Street. I've never understood why people think the idea of a little naked boy floating about with a weapon was a lovely romantic story. Also, there's not enough scrutiny around the nudity and his age. Isn't that a bit weird? It certainly feels weird.

Play your cards right, get a bit of luck and falling in love can be the most overwhelmingly brilliant thing in your life, but the stakes and emotions are high when it comes to dating, which is probably why it's so hard to navigate. Remember: There are a lot of bellends out there. I've been the bellend and I've also been bellended. None of us are entirely innocent. That's how it works. We've all behaved badly, some worse than others of course, but love makes us act irrationally, out of character and – more often than we'd care to admit – like complete lunatics.

No one warned me about the horrors of dating, though weirdly I think a certain amount of naivety is good for us because without going through it, you'll never find the good ones. Of course, the tricky thing is that the 'good ones' can become the 'bad ones' and even more annoyingly (but rarely), the 'bad ones' can also become the 'good ones'. And then they can go bad again without any warning. No one prepares you for it, but maybe no one can. I'm going to try to prepare *you* though. It's dangerous to pick apart how you've behaved in the past because a lot of it was unconscious behaviour and it just 'happened'. But I have done a lot of deep thinking about what my intentions were in my late teens, twenties and then into my thirties. Sometimes I think I spent way too long obsessing over finding love and finding a partner than I really should have. And probably that energy and brain space would have been put to better use prioritising my friendships, my family and my hobbies. Essentially, I think I made it all too important. Perhaps that was societal pressure where love and marriage are held as the Holy Grail of adulthood. But perhaps in my case, it's just how it was supposed to go. Maybe a big part of my development into being a 'grown-up' was working out who I fancied, who I liked hanging out with and who I fell in love with. Falling in and out of love is famously something you can't control much, but I do think I could have been a little smarter with some of my decisions.

I'm almost certain that being at a boys' secondary school stunted my emotional growth in this area and if I'd have been around girls on a daily basis a) I wouldn't have been so scared of them and b) I would have had a few more girl friends (and by that I mean friends that were girls). I didn't really have any until sixth form (which was mixed) and a mere two years later I was at university. It all happened very quickly and I was overwhelmed. I had my first proper girlfriend in sixth form who was brilliant and amazing but I didn't know what I was doing at all. Neither did she, probably, but girls are just smarter and better so she just always seemed way more together than I was. Those early relationships are all part of the process. At the time, they are the biggest thing in your life but, cynically, if they're nurturing and fun, they help you grow, they probably increase your confidence in talking to other people you're attracted to as well. The problem I had for a few years was working out that 99 per cent of the time a girl came to talk to me, it was just to be nice and potentially become a friend. It's hideously embarrassing to look back at the times I misread a situation. During my first year of university, I remember being a terrifying mixture of overwhelmed and underprepared. Nowhere near cerebrally developed enough to realise when a girl wanted to just be pleasant and when they wanted to maybe touch your willy. I hate admitting that. But this is how it should be. You should be acutely aware of how incredibly mortifying it is to be a human at all times. When you come to terms with this, life becomes simpler and weirdly more enjoyable. It's also the only way to learn. We are fallible, flawed, weird, horny mammals. Humans are capable of many great things but we're also capable of truly tooth-aching cringe. How can it be that we built the Great Wall of China, channelled a tunnel under the seabed to France and invented the wheel (for ancient chariots, not Michael McIntyre), and yet we still crumble into several pathetic pieces because the girl you fancied for ages gets off with someone else?

Of course I matured, eventually, calmed down and as the three years went on I made some amazing girl friends at university, but for a long time afterwards – into my twenties and even into my thirties – I let dating and relationships occupy way too much real estate in my brain. I also gave the idea of finding 'the one' way too much importance. I suppose this was partly to do with my own lack of self-esteem and a learnt belief that you're a more complete adult if you're validated by a partner. This of course isn't the case, but it's something that was niggling at me for years. These ideas of what 'success' or 'happiness' are simply can't work for everyone. Some people are really happy on their own – forever. And that's fine. There isn't a one-size-fits-all template.

All the best for the future

The most important thing, which took me a while to learn, was making sure you're OK on your own first so you minimise the risk of fucking up someone else's life while trying to make sense of yours. But how do you do that without having some dodgy relationships along the way? It's an imprecise science because you can do all the best 'work' on yourself and still meet someone who wrecks your life, but you'll recover a lot better if you have a strong sense of yourself.

I have been incredibly lucky in my dating life. I've met and fallen in love with some brilliant people who have (on the whole) enriched my life massively and I hope at least a couple of them feel the same about me (needy). But that journey has also been punctuated by heartache. In hindsight, even if the way some of those relationships ended was horrible or messy or took too long, all of them were right to end. There were ones that ended abruptly, some that petered out, some that took ages and some that went – came back – went again – came back and went again. Oh, and then came back. I had one of those in my late twenties and it was one of the most hurtful for me. I lost my sense of self almost entirely. Friends noticed a change in me, I lost confidence in my work and who I was as a person, and doubted everything I was and had done. It was a bizarre couple of years. I could sit here and blame the person and that would be really easy – and quite fun to bitch someone out. But it would also be unfair. Taking accountability is a very uncomfortable lesson to learn but I've worked hard at it over the last ten years and I've reached the conclusion that it was a classic case of something that lasted way longer than it should have done. Mainly because we were both immature and just desperate for it to work despite deep down knowing that it was a dreadful idea. We just weren't ready for each other. We weren't ready for anyone. And it took us ages to realise and it caused a lot of hurt for both of us. All these relationships are important, though. You learn a lot about yourself in each one. I always think it's dangerous to create the narrative that a break-up is a failure because what does that do for you? It just makes you feel like shit. My wise old friend Louis once said to me after a break-up, 'It's sad but no one died and you'll both get over it.' And, look, at the time of writing, I'm still alive and to the best of my knowledge, so is she.

Timing is something smug people who are giving advice talk about a lot. And yes, there's the literal timing of two people being single, which is preferable and important but more than anything, the slightly more nuanced version of that is timing in terms of emotional availability. It's always really sad when things are going really well but there's a little something that terminates it. Nothing massive, but still something significant and there's no going back from it. You're both not quite at the same stage of either fully getting over someone else, or you're not ready to move in or meet their friends or whatever. It's a shame when that happens but it is for the best. It always is. My main bit of big brotherly advice is that if it's sapping your energy and it's just not working despite really trying, it's not going to happen. It's so difficult, though. Your head's saying one thing, your heart another and let's be frank, your genitals are saying something else altogether. It's difficult to know what to do for the best sometimes because sex is really great fun. It's also extra hard (pardon the pun) if they're really fit.

What I do know is that when Bella and I arrived in each other's lives, we were completely ready to explore what it could become. I'd spent a really good amount of quality time on my own, rebuilding myself, travelling, getting fit, starting some exciting new work things and spending time with the friends I'd neglected. And for the first time in a long time, I wasn't looking for a relationship – and there we go. It happened. And it was, and still is, the best thing ever. As soon as we met, I realised that she had also been through some stuff and similarly had spent the preceding few years working on herself. She'd remembered what it was that made her great, dated some people, did some fun things and worked out how to come back from 'the stuff' she'd been through.

The 'stuff' turned out to be ... A DIVORCE! Wow! A *real* grown-up. Proper adult things! Even me being exposed to the details of it all taught me a lesson: it's not the end of the world if you get divorced. You don't die, life is long and you can still find happiness, no matter what came before.

I'm Not Coming to Your Wedding in Greece

I'd never dated a divorcee. I remember this being a bit weird at first and I'm not sure why. I suppose there's a shame associated with divorce and there really shouldn't be. A break-up isn't a failure. Break-ups are sad for sure, sometimes messy, definitely painful and unsettling, but they're not failures. We're all mad. Humans malfunction, we're not perfect and these things happen – and statistically quite often, too. Almost half of all marriages end in divorce so it's a genuine achievement if you can keep it together forever. It doesn't make you less of a catch if you're divorced but maybe when I met Bella, that's something that crossed my mind briefly. Just because of society and how frowned upon divorce has historically been. Any prejudices I had left my mind as soon as I met her because it was immediately clear that she was completely amazing.

Interestingly, the idea of marriage hadn't really featured loudly in my life plans. Not out of choice, nor a deeply held rejection of the idea of it, but I somehow couldn't imagine it. It felt like something *other* people did. People who were more together and grown up than I was. I was surprised that Bella wanted to get married again and even more surprised that she was the one who proposed to *me*. And I'm so glad she did. I am proudly Bella's second husband. The current Mr Mackie. She first got married when she was 28 and it was basically a disaster. I'm glad about that and I'm very grateful to the bloke that fucked it up the first time round – and so is she, I assume.

In the process of writing this book, I've realised that my favourite philosopher is Rebecca Lucy Taylor, aka the singer Self Esteem. This is her third mention in the book. In her song 'I Do This All the Time' is the lyric that your wedding isn't 'the biggest day of your life' because 'all the days you get to have are big'. I couldn't agree more. Of course you should have a magical day where all your favourite people (and a couple of twats from work you had to invite) will be in the same place and you'll really feel the love. But remember, you'll have plenty of great ordinary days where you'll probably be happier, less stressed about table plans and whether your nan's going to say outdated offensive things she's read in the *Daily Express* to the bride's family. Your wedding day shouldn't be the best day of your life. Of course it should be exciting because it's the beginning of hopefully a really fun new chapter, but how depressing to think that you've just had your best day! The inference is that it's all downhill from here, babes! Much like Christmas Day, there's just too much pressure on the day itself. It can't possibly live up to some of the stress, strain and logistical planning that goes into it.

We also need to make sure we separate the wedding from the marriage itself. Make sure you're not just in love with the idea of THE BIG DAY and you've also given serious thought to the rest of it. It's hopefully the start of a long road and you're going to learn pretty quickly that when the marquee has been taken down, the vomit mopped up and the deposit lost, it's just the two of you.

Alone together. Forever. Until one of you dies. Or sleeps with their personal trainer. It's easy to get fixated on the 'getting married' bit as the destination, much like when people decide to have a baby. How many people do you know that have said, 'Oh, I'd love to have a baby!' while not really stopping to consider whether they're fully signed up and ready to be a parent. Forevermore. Wanting a baby and wanting to be a parent are two slightly different things. Same with wanting to get married and wanting to *be* married to someone. There's a difference.

I really don't agree that there's only one person you're meant to be with. That's heading towards fairy tale nonsense. There was a thing going around TikTok not long ago saying that you marry the person you're with when you want to get married. This is an oversimplification and very general but I think there's a truth in it. It takes some of the magical mystery away but life isn't always magical and mysterious. It's beautifully mundane and functional sometimes, which is perhaps too far the other way from the 'fairy tale' idea; the truth is probably somewhere between the two. Life shouldn't be a fairy tale. That's weird, unrealistic and, ironically, quite boring. Unpredictable is good sometimes.

Bella and I had been going out for seven months when she asked me to marry her. WHAT?! The *woman* asking the *man* to marry her?! I loved it. I thought she was mad. (She *is* mad.) I was about to go off and do a big challenge for Comic Relief where I was set to climb the three peaks (Snowdon, Scafell Pike and Ben Nevis) and cycle between them over a week in February 2018. This was a ludicrous challenge and something I was nervous about. But, it turns out, not as nervous as Bella was. We went out for a goodbye dinner at Bottega Prelibato in Shoreditch (it's very nice) and as I looked up from my minestrone soup, Bella was in tears. She later told me it was a mixture of her being worried I was going to die on this stupid challenge and extreme anxiety that I would say no to the question she was about to ask me. 'I was wondering if you wanted to get married?' she said. I momentarily stopped slurping, 'Yeah, of course I do,' I replied, 'definitely.' I went straight back to slurping my soup because I hadn't realised this was a proper proposal and she was asking if I wanted to get married to *her* and *now*. My mind was on carb-loading and wondering what the weather in Snowdonia was doing for the first climb, so I wasn't perhaps as effusive as I should have been. I eventually realised what she meant and obviously said yes immediately. But in Bella's dramatic retelling of this, I didn't. And also, apparently, I muttered something about not telling anyone until the challenge was done. She still holds it against me that I gave off the impression I wasn't keen. In hindsight, I should have been much more aware of the magnitude of this for her. She had already had one marriage go tits up and here she was being vulnerable yet so sure of her feelings that she wanted to go again. She was terrified too that I was going to die on the challenge and wanted to make sure I knew how much she loved me. She also wanted to hitch her train to the wagon as I was to return from that adventure a national treasure. And although it was totally unexpected and I was preoccupied about whether I'd packed enough layers, it was perfect because it wasn't 'perfect'. But this is it, right? This is what I'm talking about. Not everything has to be a fairy tale. Nothing is perfect or flawless. It was very in keeping with our relationship. Sweet, loving but disorganised, a bit shonky and accompanied by lots of wine. It now also makes a sweet little story and the main thing is she asked me, which was one of the happiest moments of my life, and we haven't looked back since. Also, I didn't die on the mountains. And she *did* get to marry the national treasure.

Something I was really keen to push through when we got married was that I wanted to really think about what the wedding day was going to be like. She'd already had a big white church wedding and I really didn't want that. I wanted to make sure it reflected who we are. There's an enormous temptation to get carried away and convince yourselves that the classic church wedding you see on the telly is what you *should* have. That's amazing if you *do* want that, of course. But it *can't* possibly be to everyone's taste. I didn't want all the groomsmen to be dressed in the same bad suit, Bella didn't want to be arsed with going shopping to get all the bridesmaids' dresses fitted. I didn't fancy traipsing round endless barns in the countryside looking at their wedding packages and menus only to realise that once you'd had your magical day and spent enough money to buy a decent second-hand Porsche 911 (I checked), you have to clear out because it's someone else's turn tomorrow. I wanted to do anything I could to make sure we disguised the fact that we were doing one of the most basic things you can do. I didn't just want to go through the motions, but it's an easy trap to fall into. We are all guilty of acting from a place of 'oh, I should do that' rather than from a place of 'I want to do that'.

I also get this feeling with funerals. I vividly remember my grandad's cremation back in the early noughties. It was the first one I'd been to and I hated it. Obviously. But the bleak memory I have is of watching the next bunch of mourners waiting to come into the room as we were being ushered out the side door. As I looked back, I saw plumes of smoke coming from the chimney as the next hearse pulled in. The unthinking routineness of it is what I hated so much. A conveyor belt of corpses. All orchestrated by Ellie, the caller I mentioned earlier, I guess. Grandad was given a time slot like he was booking a squash court down at a leisure centre. It felt so far away from the fantastic old man I knew. The man that taught me so many brilliant things, encouraged my love of gardening, making up games, playing darts and fixing things was reduced, like all those old men before him and after him, to grandad dust. There has to be a better way of doing things. I can't bear the thought of going like that.

Bella and I thought about what we'd like to do for our wedding day, who we'd like to have there and where we wanted it in an attempt to make it as 'us' as possible. Why would we suddenly become characters play-acting a wedding like it was an episode of *Bridgerton*? Lots of people love this idea and that's great, but only if it's what you want. A wedding can be the perfect excuse to put on some over-the-top costumes and play-act being a princess or whatever but instead, we became insufferable in a different way and had a very modest ceremony at Camden Registry Office. I wore a very un-wedding green snazzy suit; Bella wore an incredible bright yellow dress. It was informal – God, Jesus and all that lot didn't feature, my niece, who was 11 at the time, accompanied me down the aisle, while Bella's sister walked her down and we played 'The Ballad of Barry and Freda' by one of our favourite comedians, Victoria Wood. The famous lyrics are 'Let's do it, let's do it …' etc. It's funny. You should listen to it now. Our dads read out a couple of short poems and we were wed! That was it. A done deal.

All this was followed by a reception in a pub around the corner and then we went on to a nice restaurant for a big dinner and an even bigger piss-up with about 100 people locked in for dancing and drunkenness until the early hours. Nestled in there were some amazing (and, crucially, *short*) speeches from Bella's mum; her best man, Archie; and my best man, Will. And that was it. Everyone got hammered, my uncle fell down the stairs, we had a big cake made out of various cheeses and it was really great and exactly what we wanted. And Uncle Dave survived.

I'm sure some of the guests would have preferred a night away in a barn in Sussex. But our wedding day wasn't for them. It was for us. There is extraordinary pressure from parents, other busy-body family and friends to have the wedding *they* want you to have but here's a good thing to remember – have the wedding the two of you want to have. Use your imagination. Or if you don't have an imagination and you really couldn't give a shit what it's like, just copy someone else. Oh, and if you feel pressure to invite someone because you think you should, don't. Life's too short to look out at the congregation as you make your vows and see your friend's weird new sweaty boyfriend looking down at his phone checking to see how Preston North End are getting on in the FA Cup third round. You don't want to see them there. They don't want to be there. And you don't want them there either.

It's time now to sing the Unpopular Opinion theme tune. Those unfamiliar with my work on *The Radio 1 Breakfast Show* won't know what this is but it's pretty self-explanatory. Listeners come on the show and say something that will have caused outrage among their friends. And I'm about to annoy so many of you.

Come and give us your Unpopular Opinion, something up tillnow that you've been scared to say …

Greg …!

You shouldn't be doing a destination wedding.

I'm sorry but no one really wants to go to it. The intention might well be honourable but your friends will open the invitation, see the words Amalfi Coast and sigh. It's true. I'm sorry. It might seem like a nice idea, but in reality, it's not. It's a massive pain in the arse. As soon as we read the invitation, even though it's a beautiful part of the world, all we think about is, *I haven't got enough annual leave left for this. Who's going to look after the kids/ dog? What airport is it near? Fucking hell, flights will be so expensive at that time of the year.* If you were to put a gun to your guests' heads (which I wouldn't recommend) and ask if they'd rather the wedding was around the corner so they could save a few hundred quid and slink off back to their own bed by the time ties start becoming headbands, I bet most of them would say yes. Caveat! If one of you is originally from the place you're forcing us all to go to, I think that's OK. One of my best friends is half Swedish so we all went to Stockholm a few years ago and she got married in the same church as her grandparents and we had a great weekend exploring a beautiful part of the world with her as a guide. I get that. I'm not a complete monster. That's lovely. A few years ago, a group of us went to a wedding in Provence and on arriving at this beautiful vineyard after eight long hours of travelling, I asked the bride and groom about their connection to the region. There wasn't one. They'd never been to the vineyard. They'd never been to *any* vineyard. This wasn't just their first time in Provence, it was their first trip *to France*. No connection to the place at all. Nothing. It's mad when you look around at the congregation and it's just a collection of people who all live within a 10-mile radius of one another who've spent hundreds of pounds flying a thousand miles to hang out in France for a few hours before making their way back to the airport Novotel to fly home the next day.

I almost got back in the car and drove off. Don't gamble with our lives like that.

The other exception to my flat refusal to go to a wedding abroad is if the bride and groom are willing to pay for all of it. And I mean all of it. Flights, accommodation, spending money, hire car, all food. Other than that, no. But here's some advice. I'm telling you this right now. And you must listen. It's absolutely OK not to go. There are a maximum of about two lovely enjoyable hours at a destination wedding. Two hours out of a minimum of 48. The ratios are all off. You're not a bad person for thinking these thoughts, either. You can love the people that are getting married, you can be grateful that you were there in that moment where the marriage was confirmed but you can also think that everything else around it is a complete fucking nightmare. Both things can be true. It's particularly galling too if you're one of the friends who have steered the bride or groom through the choppy waters of their past relationships. I wouldn't put my friends through it. They've been through enough. I'm embarrassed by the amount of quality time I've wasted with my amazing friends, moaning to them about my love life. If you're close enough to have been invited abroad then you almost certainly know intimate details of Laura and Mark's rocky patch. Or the guy at work that Laura nearly had a thing with 'in the early days', or Mark's ex that he still sees a bit because they go to the same gym. We can't all pretend everything's perfect just because we're in Pisa. It's a collective madness.

It's just a lot of effort and life is already a lot of effort anyway. It's full of logistics at the best of times without having to sort this out. You'll kid yourself that you can 'make it into a holiday', but that's not ideal, is it? You're in a stunning part of the world but you'd rather go there on your own terms. You're on holiday but not on holiday. It's a trick. Like when school tries to make you think they're treating you like adults during A levels and you get a few free periods a week. You've got no lessons but you've still got to sit around at school in your uniform. Same with a destination wedding. You're trapped in wedding prison and the congregation are the other inmates. The prison uniform is linen suits and sunglasses. Prisoners will all meet at 5pm in the garden for Aperols and awkward chat about the weather and hire cars. 'Europcar were very good actua—' *Oh, SHUT UP, Ian!*

The brass neck on people to demand that their closest friends all attend their special weekend (WEEK, sometimes!). How dare you? I'd feel awful about it. Tuscany obviously crossed my mind because I'm a middle-class prick and I get it, it's a lovely idea. But leave it as an idea. You're not Amal Clooney. Even if you've managed to save up and are happy to write the cost off, no one else will be able to. Or want to. You're forcing people to have a holiday *for you*. Think how much you value your precious holiday allowance. It's evil to expect this of everyone you supposedly love. My friends would have hated me. All of them silently and furiously booking flights. Thinking about what to wear. Is it going to be hot? What's my most Italian-looking suit? How the fuck do you take a long dress on Ryanair? No thanks. Instead, Bella and I had a perfect day getting married in London, so 85 per cent of the guests could make it there fairly easily and – crucially – get home when they'd (and we'd) had enough.

One of the huge problems with weddings in general is that you barely get to have any meaningful conversation or interaction with the bride or groom. They're busy. They're untouchable on their special day. These people you've probably known for your entire life are suddenly A-listers. For that night, the most famous people in the world. You can't believe they're talking to you, briefly. 'Hey! You're the guys from the church and the old car!' And presumably you're there because you love one or both of them dearly. It's always the way at weddings that the bride and groom have to spend most of their time with the people they least wanted to invite. If you're close to either of them, forget it. They know you'll be OK, you see them all the time. But weird Tim from work who doesn't know anyone else is way more needy so they have to hang around with him talking about their shit boss or how lucky they've been with the weather. Meanwhile, you're having to put in a proper shift with their university banter brigade. 'Oh guys, remember Soph during freshers?' No, I don't. And I don't want to either. Also, get over freshers' week, you're 30 and your hair's going at the temples. Sophie used to slag you off to me (her *real* friend) every holiday when we all met up at home in the Black Lion. Side note, while I'm ranting, anyone over the age of 25 that regularly brings up how great school or university was is boring.

All of those things are just about manageable if the wedding is close to home in familiar surroundings, but if you're 1,500 miles away and you've only got Luton airport on a Sunday night to look forward to, it's a living nightmare. Transplant a wedding out of the UK and you're just on holiday with a load of strangers. You're standing around all hot and drunk in a beautiful part of the world, trying to find common ground with the ultimate frisbee bellends, unable to hang out with the people you've come to celebrate. If you're thinking about a destination wedding, don't do it. Don't put everyone through it. It's unkind. Plus it's really embarrassing if you end up getting divorced. There's a lot of pressure to make good our investments. Thinking about it, we should be reimbursed if it all goes to shit. Can guests do prenups? Can you take out wedding insurance to get the cost of the present and the flights back if they don't go the distance? Are weddings ATOL protected? Oh, and in case you're wondering, the same rules apply to hen and stag dos abroad. I'm not going.

So, after all that moaning, is getting married any good? Does it feel any different? It does for me, yeah. I love it. I feel so calm in my marriage. It's the best thing in my life. The most important thing in my life. A kind, loving, fun base that I get to hang out at. But a base that we feel happy leaving to go and dive into work or disappear off with friends knowing full well that this amazing, intangible sanctum is there when I return. I feel simultaneously free to explore who I am and what I can achieve but also rooted firmly with a person who I trust with everything. My marriage with Bella has supplied me with the missing paints I needed to colour in the bits of my life I couldn't quite see or understand. I haven't mentioned it to her in these terms. I'll wait for her to read the book. But my guess (and my hope) is that she feels exactly the same way about it. If not, she can always get divorced again.

Always Meet Your Heroes

Before you get married, however, you have to find out as much as you can about the person you're preparing to spend the rest of your life with. 'We're so alike!' or 'We just love all the same stuff!' was something that always seemed to be celebrated whenever I saw couples declaring their love for each other in TV shows and films. It's nice to have shared interests, but I've always found it a bit creepy when you realise someone has essentially just married themselves. I've always thought it was way more important to both *hate* similar things. Think about your friends. You probably bond most when you're slagging something or someone off. Nothing brings us together more than a common enemy. For me and Bella when we started chatting in 2016/17, it was the age of Piers Morgan, Farage and Trump. Lots of good stuff to go at there.

It's disconcerting when you meet people who don't have strong views about anything in particular. Who and what do you LOVE? Who do you HATE? Who are your idols? These are all really decent first-date questions, because you can tell a lot about a person from their answers. It's useful so you can get out early if they adore something you detest, isn't it? Nothing worse than falling in love with someone and then finding out they once took a day off work to visit the Spud Van or finding out their dream is to get married at Disney World and their favourite comedian is a racist one. Back to idols then. Whether it's Fireman Sam (the firefighter), Graeme Hick (the cricketer) or Larry David for being perhaps the funniest person alive, my life has been littered with them and hopefully yours has too. Some idols hold a special place in your heart, others will come and go as you get older. Much like the League of Friends, some idols will go up in your estimation and some will go down. Some will disgrace themselves, some will even be cancelled (take your pick) and need to be replaced. New characters will pop up because their performance in a recent film wowed you (Mikey Madison in *Anora*), a book they wrote lit up a holiday you had (Michael Palin's recent diaries), an album they made got under your skin (the latest one from Lorde and again Self Esteem – fourth mention now) or a TikTokker inspired you to fall back in love with the things you loved as a kid (Francis Bourgeois and his trains).

There are loads of people I looked up to as a kid and well into my teenage years that I still think fondly about. Of course, some of them have fallen by the wayside in terms of impact, for instance, Mr Blobby doesn't feature much in my day-to-day life these days, but there are a couple that are still regularly very much in my thoughts and, bizarrely, now feature in my actual life. It's a real privilege getting to spend time with some of the most famous people in the world and I never lose that sense of excitement when I meet them. Interviewing celebrities often feels like a weird fever dream because I'm normally sitting in the studio – a place where I feel so comfortable and happy – and then suddenly an A-lister walks in and contractually has to spend 30 minutes pretending that this is the only place in the world they want to be. I feel great pressure to make sure we get a good interview that the listeners like, and often that makes me nervous at the beginning, but it's rare that I get so awed by anyone that I panic about forming even the most basic sentences. I'm often asked about who makes me star-struck and I can think of only two people where this has happened in my career, and they're about as disparate as you could get. One of them is Dwayne 'The Rock' Johnson and the other is Michael 'The Nicest Man on Earth' Palin.

Palin came first, so let's start there. Before I realised he was part of the most successful comedy group of all time, Monty Python, I knew him as the nice funny man who went around the world in 80 days in his hit BBC One series *Around the World in 80 Days*. The idea of the show was that he'd follow the fictitious voyage of a character named Phileas Fogg from Jules Verne's 1872 novel of the same name. Much like Phileas, Palin decided to do the journey without using planes but with the addition of a documentary crew in tow. I still watch it at least once a year because it's utterly brilliant. For example, on my waste day! We see Michael daringly zip around the world on rickety boats on the Danube, squeezing onto over-booked trains through India and at one point even riding a camel as he traverses the Egyptian desert. Throughout his travels, he's never once condescending to either the viewer or the locals, and along the way he showed millions of us other parts of the world we'd never heard of and now, due to most of the world being at war, places we'll likely never see. And he always did it kindly, knowledgeably and humorously. He has had a profound impact on me through my life and, looking back, the way he stayed curious throughout the whole thing and made the show about everyone else but him inspired me hugely. I wouldn't have started hosting things and acting at school if it wasn't for him. It sparked an interest in other people and how they live their lives. Michael Palin finds people interesting – not for any cynical or nefarious reason but because he always wants to learn something new or find a new perspective.

Where does The Rock fit into this then? Well, he too loves meeting people, although he'd call it 'pressing the flesh'. He loves travelling around and spreading the good word of Dwayne Johnson, entertaining people and making sure they have a nice time. There are clearly some stark differences between the two men but surely there's a lot of common ground.

	Michael Palin	The Rock
Height	1.78m	1.93m
Weight	65kg	120kg – he eats a lot. That's a lot of eggs.
Famous catchphrases	'No one expects the Spanish Inquisition!' 'Ni!' 'I have a vewy gweat fwiend in Wome called Biggus Dickus!'	'If ya smellllll … what The Rock … is cookin'' 'Know your role, jabroni, and shut your mouth' 'Just bring it'
Finishing move	Slapping someone around the face with a fish	The best one is the Rock Bottom, or the People's Elbow. The Rock Bottom is better.
Favourite book	*The Old Man and the Sea* by Ernest Hemingway	*The Rock Says …* by The Rock
Shoe size	8	14 – he's definitely got a special shoe guy, hasn't he?
Age	82	53
Net worth	£20 million	£800 million

OK, there aren't many obvious similarities, I admit (apart from having silly catchphrases, which is perhaps part of the reason I was drawn to them). They both absolutely love making people smile – albeit in different ways; I've never seen Michael Palin Rock Bottom someone through a table and similarly, I've never seen The Rock sleep on bags of rice on a local man's dhow, sailing from Dubai to India over several days while suffering from intense diarrhoea and only having an open-air latrine to deal with and *still* remaining charming and funny. Obviously The Rock wouldn't need a boat. He'd swim.

As a child, you pick and choose the bits of your idols that appeal to you. I loved Michael's stoicism, kindness, sense of community and upholding of civic duties by 'mucking in'. This spirit runs through his travel shows but I also adore his unwavering passion for silliness. He's always thoughtful and intelligent but he doesn't take things or himself too seriously. He's comfortable making himself look daft in order to get a laugh, and he always commits to the task at hand, even if the task is absurd. *This* is where they're similar. They commit to 'the bit'. The Rock described himself as 'The Most Electrifying Man in All Entertainment', and that's hard to argue with but also incredibly hard to live up to – and yet he does! His confidence bursts through the screen, the crowd erupts whenever his entrance music hits. He's loud and brash but also smart and funny when interacting with the crowd and he's also able to perform *so* skilfully in the ring. The most boring thing in the world is when people say 'yeah, but wrestling's fake'. Of course it is, dickhead, but it doesn't mean it's not really difficult to train and stay fit for, choreograph and pull off *live*. It can be incredible drama because at the heart of it all is storytelling, and The Rock is one of the best in-ring storytellers ever. It helps to think of it as a form of dancing. *Strictly Come Dancing* but they hit each other over the head with steel chairs at the end of the paso doble. Not a bad idea for a format. The Rock is tough and strong, but the acting and talent required to pace the fight, come back just when you think he's down, get the crowd on side when he needs it and also nail all the moves is extraordinary. I was captivated by his charisma and swagger and his showmanship got me hooked to the entertainment industry (albeit in very different ways from Michael). I loved the scale of the show – the pyro, the lighting, the nonsense, really! That's what it is: wonderful nonsense! That's really where these two intersect. Nonsense is what draws me in, always. Python, Harry Hill, Vic and Bob, *The Big Breakfast*, Victoria Wood, *The Fast Show*, Dawn French, Alan Partridge, Chris Morris. It's all brilliantly silly.

The first time I met Michael Palin, I panicked. He'd been booked as a surprise guest on my Radio 1 drivetime show and was ushered into the studio mid-link. I didn't know what to do with myself. I blurted out a word salad about how I had derailed our family holiday to make my parents queue up with 13-year-old me to see him at a bookshop in New York when he was signing copies of his debut novel, *Hemingway's Chair*. I told him about how I obsessively read his beautifully kept diaries and repeatedly rewatched *Around the World in 80 Days*, all the time desperately trying not to creep him out too much. When I eventually calmed down, we had a lovely chat and he couldn't have been more charming and refreshingly normal. He hasn't bought into his celebrity or his legacy. He's very much focused on doing interesting work and having an enjoyable life. By all accounts, he lives a relatively ordinary life, but he has achieved extraordinary things. I love this attitude to fame; it only exists if you cultivate it. There's no right way to be a famous person, but I love the way he does it. He's rooted in the real world, in his community, in day-to-day society. I now often see him wandering around near where I live and popping to our local bookshop. Joyfully, we're now on email terms with each other and although I'm very careful not to abuse that privilege, it's been such a pleasure to get to know him a bit more. I got the opportunity to interview him at the afore-mentioned local bookshop in front of about 50 people and I also invited him onto our *Tailenders* cricket podcast and we had the most glorious 90-minute chat about cricket, music, comedy and his love for travel. He turned up on his own – no agent or manager or PR person. Just him, with his trademark satchel, armed with charming stories and anecdotes from a life and career well-lived. He was just as interested in my fellow Tailender – the greatest fast bowler ever, Jimmy Anderson – and the rest of us as we were in him. Understated and totally at ease with himself.

Dwayne Johnson is also incredibly charming and at ease with himself. My first meeting with 'The Great One' was a slightly glitz-ier affair but I still had that rush of nervous excitement that made me feel like a teenager again. It's perhaps a bit much if you end up doing this to every person that ignites that teenage excitement in you, but for the special few, I think it means you're still in touch with the old you. Or more accurately, the young you. The entire trip was promising to be bizarre even before it began because the interview was set to take place in Miami. I'm so lucky to have the life I do and it was a great adventure with a one-man crew, a very talented man called Phill, whose idea it was to do a documentary on Dwayne. A Rock-umentary, if you will. (And we did – it's on YouTube still.) The Rock was promoting the reboot of *Baywatch*, which was shit, hence being in Florida, and I decided to get fully into the spirit of things and dress up as a lifeguard for the interview. Phill had booked me in for a spray tan near the venue so I popped in there before we headed over. He thought that it would make a funny 'bit' to overdo it slightly so I'd be more orange than tanned, however, it thickened and darkened so much that at the start of the interview The Rock was jokingly concerned that I'd turned up to interview my hero in blackface. This clearly wasn't the intention. I started panicking, he started laughing at me and I knew instantly that he was up for the interview and had been briefed that I was a mega fan and definitely not a racist. He listened attentively to all my questions about his career, his impact on millions of kids around the world and his duty as an idol to do right by his fans and keep them happy. He even engaged with my lame stories of how I used to pretend to be him while wrestling my mates. I know these people have to feign interest a lot of the time, but you can usually tell when someone's putting it on. He wasn't.

With my dad's job as a headteacher, there were still some perks, one of which was that we had access to the school's sports hall and therefore the crash mats. My mates and I would go over to Enfield on a Saturday (while he went and worked) and beat each other up for a few hours. We filmed it of course, and I showed this video to The Rock. If there's a greater illustration of being in touch with your childlike joy, I'd like to see one. The circle was complete.

He was looking at the proof that I've been obsessed with him since I was 14 and he said it was *good* (apart from a weird thing I was doing with my legs).

Dwayne was back in the UK just before Christmas 2024 promoting his new festive movie *Red One*, and we had an interview scheduled in. As he approached me outside the BBC he shouted 'Buddy!', which was very nice and also appropriate as I was dressed as an elf. Before we started recording, he said, 'You know, we go back a long time, don't we? I was thinking on the way over that it's been a decade.' Now, obviously, you don't get to be The Rock without that sort of prep and attention to detail, but it's still rare. Very few A-listers are like that as they meet so many people and couldn't possibly remember everyone. So this extra effort shows that he at least cares enough to make sure people *think* he cares! He wants everyone to feel special and that in itself is a lovely way to operate. He asked me questions about the *Breakfast Show*, how I was, how life was and then we got down to the interview. He doesn't have to do that, and again, most guests don't ask you anything about yourself, but he realises what it's like to be on the receiving end of that and knows that it can make someone's day – and if you can make someone's day relatively easily, why wouldn't you?

The day we met was the morning after America had just decided they wanted a convicted felon to be its president again for another few years. He didn't give much away but thanked me for steering clear of any questions about it. He showed public support for Biden and Harris in 2020 but decided not to publicly support anyone in this election cycle. My hunch is he doesn't care much for Trump. I mean, why would he? As a child of immigrants, a

Samoan mother and African American father, he probably hates everything he stands for. Whatever his allegiances and whatever his reason for not publicly backing Harris, for the first time, I got a glimpse into the real Dwayne. A heartfelt, non-showbiz 'thank you' for not asking him about politics. I don't know what I think about incredibly famous people showing their support for politicians – I think you can argue it both ways and in any case, if Beyoncé, Taylor Swift, LeBron James and Cardi B can't make a difference (they all supported Kamala), did we really miss The Rock's endorsement? I told him about this book I'm writing and that there's half a chapter about him, at which his face lit up and he gave me a bear hug. I asked if he'd do a quote for the front of the book and he replied, 'Of course'. I've since decided to pay homage to a dead duck who resulted in me being given a doctorate, or a 'ducktorate' if you will. We said goodbye, then he got into one of the many SUVs in the convoy and was whisked off to charisma-bomb the next interviewer. I got back to Radio 1, changed out of my elf costume, wiped the lipstick off my cheeks that I'd put on to make them look rosy and began my cycle home, and as I passed the Holiday Inn, I reflected on that mad afternoon spent with my teenage idol. I started to feel a bit sad for him because as he's become one of the most famous people in the world, people don't consider that he has feelings and deep, complex thoughts. He's a highly intelligent man but I can't help but think this persona means that the real essence of Dwayne Johnson has to remain deeply hidden behind that enormous smile and even bigger biceps, the electrifying charisma and a life of pressing the flesh with people who idolise you. Maybe I'm completely wrong and maybe he is still in touch with his true self, but it struck me that whenever he goes anywhere public, he's The Rock. Basically a superhero, unable to sit quietly in a pub, impossible to get on a train and take a day trip somewhere, he can't sit and watch a football match or a concert unless he's in a VIP box. He probably doesn't do the big shop, he can't just wander round a park without someone stopping him and asking about WrestleMania. And look, he probably loves being The Rock. He has a great life, he's made more money than he knows what to do with and wherever he goes, he gets hero-worshipped. I suppose even if he didn't, he has no choice now, but I often look at really famous celebrities and think, how famous is too famous? For me, that would be too famous. Your whole life turns into the show and maybe you forget some of the things that made you, you. I wonder how in touch with his younger self The Rock is? Maybe I'll get to ask him one day.

This ode to celebrity hero-worship must come with a WARN-ING. Michael Palin and The Rock have given me a lot but this isn't necessarily a two-way relationship. The thing Palin offered me was *Around the World In 80 Days* and the thing I offered him was being an extra viewer. There is no third act here. The joy in these relationships should be one-sided. The lines have become increasingly blurred because of the internet and the chance to get noticed by your heroes. Famous people, content creators and influencers actively want us to feel like they're our friends, but they're not really. Being unaware of this carefully constructed illusion can come with a downside. Para-social relationships are very easily formed when you are enticed into buying something from a celebrity 'brand' because they've welcomed you into what they call their 'community.' You begin to imagine that this gives you some ingress into their lives, that you're entitled to more somehow.

As with everything in life, moderation and boundaries are important here because, before you know it, you're communicating or interacting with people you've never met instead of your actual friends. Instagram, Snapchat and TikTok are very deliberately designed so that the most famous people in the world appear on the same feed as your school and work friends.

Sometimes celebrities also fall into this trap of feeling like their fans are their friends. They can be so keen to curate their 'relatable' image online that they hold nothing back, and overshare as if talking to their best friends. I don't want to know *everything* about my heroes. Sometimes keeping people online at arm's length is important. If nothing else, a sense of distance helps me keep celebrities separate from my real friends and stops me from ever getting to the point where I think they owe me something in return for my adoration. We can expect too much of people in the public eye and because our relationships can be 'close', if they say the 'wrong' thing, follow the 'wrong' person or don't speak out on every issue that matters to us, we can take it as a personal affront. This is known as 'The Halo Effect' and, again, because I'm smart, I read about it in a great book by Amanda Montell called *The Age of Magical Overthinking*. It's a very good read. I recommend it. Amanda explains the idea of attributing positive traits to celebrities without even knowing them. Then, if this person that they've spent their time and energy engaging with and supporting suddenly steps out of the constructed image of them, the fan feels betrayed.

Having heroes is great in many ways, but they don't owe us anything. Yes, they want us to like them (and sometimes they want us to buy stuff from them) but they're human beings, and probably best not taken too seriously. They can be a great reminder of your childhood passions and obsessions, who you are or used to be, what you liked, what you now no longer like and maybe what you still want to be, but they're not a mirror of you.

I have complicated feelings about this. Because on the one hand, I love being people's mate on the radio and I genuinely enjoy the interactions I have with listeners as a result. But being sort of famous has made me understand that parasocial relationships can be tricky for both sides. You can get a lot from liking someone's work or feeling like someone in the public eye represents or reflects you in a certain way. But these connections shouldn't replace traditional friendships. The great thing about my job and others like mine is that we have the joy of being a conduit for people to find like-minded friends, and I love that we create a safe space to encourage that on the radio. It brings me so much joy and makes the job feel meaningful.

Whoever your heroes are or were will probably have shaped you in some way. Your relationship with the people you idolised will evolve as you grow up – maybe you won't care about Fireman Sam in your thirties – but it's still important to stay connected to the feelings they provoked in you, even if you don't obsess over the person in the same way. I view some of the people I became a fan of as a child as a sort of guide you take with you along the way. Their presence through their music or art or comedy is, at best, a constant through whatever life throws at you, and can serve as a distraction or even more profoundly, a comfort. You'll probably laugh at some of the obsessions you used to have, some of the trips you took to see them in concert, the hours spent outside the stage door just to catch a glimpse. These things are brilliant and I don't think we truly appreciate their importance. I hate it when people dismiss teenage pop music fans, for example. It's amazing to feel an affinity with something or someone, to feel like you belong somewhere. I remember talking to someone at the time One Direction started to blow up globally and they said, 'Yeah, but it's just a load of young girls that fancy them.' It was such an obnoxious thing to say. This person completely missed the point of fandom. It offers people a safe space to explore their own personality when perhaps they don't feel comfortable sharing the things they worry about in person or with their families; these could be anxieties around sexuality, identity, growing up or dating. On a very simple level, fandom can offer friendship and community if you haven't found your tribe in real life yet. These early experiences where you look up to others start to shape who you are and who you become. Those young fans grow up into adults who might go on to change the world, and those early passions and urges need to be treated with respect. They're all valid, even if a world-weary adult finds it embarrassing. The teenagers who mass fainted at Beatles concerts grew up to run the world. Let people have heroes, just remember you won't actually end up marrying your favourite celebrity. Well, unless you're Hailey Bieber. Get that bag, hunni!

Are You That Bloke off the Thing?

I prefer to think of myself as fairly 'well known' rather than a celebrity. Being well known means that a lot of people get to know who you are and you notice it immediately. Mine is the first voice millions of people hear every day and so people get to know it well and in turn, they get to know you well too. Both of those things are a privilege and it honestly never gets old being at the whim of the *Breakfast Show* listeners every morning, fielding the calls, reading the messages and being a ringleader for whatever mad thing they seem to grab on to that morning. The fact that people care enough to interact with the stuff we come up with is something I never take for granted and my time on that show will live so fondly in my memory forever. I've made it sound like I'm leaving. I'm not, as far as I know, leaving for a while yet.

But being thought of as a 'celebrity' really cringes me out. Part of why radio appealed to me is that you get to entertain lots of people but you're not really a celebrity. That said, if I hated 'being known' so much, I could have chosen a job that was completely anonymous, so there's definitely a part of me that wants to be heard or liked or maybe even adored. Perhaps that's one to unpack with the therapist. With radio, though, you can dip your toe into the apparently glossy showbiz world then report back to tell the listeners that actually it's a pile of shit and not as glamorous as it appears. With radio, you're a friend to the listeners, and when you return home after the show, you're one of them again. Being a bit famous is still weird sometimes. I've got used to hearing the whispered version of my name now; it happens as people walk past and maybe think it's me. I can hear the mumble of it being said in the distance. Let me tell you this, from being on the receiving end of it, when we see a famous person, we're all much louder than we realise. Here's a fun exercise: say my name without moving your mouth. That's what I hear sometimes on the street or in a pub. I do it all the time if I see someone famous in the wild. There's a lot of them knocking around north London. I saw the actor Simon Farnaby in a pub the other day. He's the very funny man from *Ghosts*, *Horrible Histories* and *Paddington*. I turned to my mates and reported back immediately and probably loudly to the point that he would have almost certainly heard me. So, I get it. A bit like seeing one of your teachers on the high street on a Saturday morning, seeing a famous person out and about is a treat and it's weird when you realise they have an actual life.

I can't imagine how awful it must be to have reached *real* fame, though. You know that level of fame where the entire room would fall silent as you walked in? The level of fame where they're selling cardboard masks of your faces in those tourist tat shops. The Rock, basically. Imagine not being able to go to your favourite pub or sit on a train without everyone trying to take a photo of you. I genuinely think I've got the perfect amount of fame. Before everything on the radio was filmed, you'd have to do some serious digging to work out what your favourite presenters even looked like. The internet, and particularly social media, has decreased my chances of remaining anonymous quite significantly but it's really not an issue. And in any case, I think I've massively benefitted from the stuff I've done online as it helps build up a literal picture of who you're listening to. I'm lucky that I have a level of recognition where people are incredibly nice to me if they see me somewhere. I'm not everywhere or unavoidable, I don't think. If anything, I go the opposite way. I don't go to too many things. Mainly because they're boring and full of annoying famous people but also because I'd rather be with my mates or Bella or my dog or just in the bath.

I'm lucky enough to get asked onto lots of fun things, and that in itself is a privilege, I realise. But I've been at this for long enough now to know what I don't want to do just for the sake of a bit of profile raising. The odd appearance on a panel show or *Taskmaster* or *Bake Off* is a real treat, but I'm also lucky that I *have* a job that keeps me in the minds of everyone so I don't need to constantly appear on everything. *Strictly*'s an interesting one. I have been asked a few times to go on it now and I've very politely said no. It's incredibly flattering to be invited on the biggest show in the country. And about ten years ago, I got really close to saying yes. There are two reasons that people go on big reality shows and I'd love it if just one person was honest about it one year. 'I'm doing it for the money, babes!' or 'I just want to raise the profile a bit to be honest! Everyone's forgotten who I am and I haven't worked for a while!' Don't fall for the 'Oh I really want to learn a new skill!' line. Go and take dance lessons at the village hall then. 'I want to conquer my fear of heights and creepy crawlies!' Well, you don't need Ant and Dec to be there while you do it, do you dear. Be honest, you're doing it so you can host your own ITV game show in a couple of years and that's fine! Don't pretend you're doing a reality show just so you can wave to your kids through the telly when the judges are slagging off your salsa.

Those shows give you quite intense tabloid fame very quickly. And I've always thought it was a bit of a dangerous game. I don't love that level of uncontrolled exposure because you can become fodder and it can be horribly intrusive and can interrupt the lovely simple connection you might already have with your audience. I try my best to avoid that level of press attention just for being on TV or *being* a celebrity. I'm sure Radio 1 would love it if I was splashed all over the Sidebar of Shame every day but I would be really sad and stressed about it. Being mentioned on the Sidebar of Shame for trying to get Alison Hammond into space, though? Jackpot! I guess as much as possible, I want to be talked about for the work that I do, not the behind-the-scenes drama of a reality show. I don't feel the need to be 'on' the whole time, if that makes sense? As I've got older, I've taken just as much pleasure from making the thing as I have from hosting the thing or at least being the centre of it. The idea of being content with creating the thing and not having to be the centre of attention doesn't always track with the social media phenomenon of being an 'influencer'. 'YouTuber' is still really high on the list of careers kids aspire to. But instead of rolling my eyes, moaning and sounding like the oldest man in the world, I recognise that that's not new. Or particularly surprising. I vividly remember even when I was a teenager that there was some study or other proclaiming that the world was fucked because all kids wanted to do was *be famous*. That desire has been around for as long as TV and film have existed. But I think a smarter question to ask is, 'Famous for what?' Do a thing really well and you might get well known for it. Get good at something you're passionate about and use that as the driving force, not 'I just want to be famous.' When I was eight, I wanted to be a TV presenter because that's what I was watching and what appealed to me. A few years later I discovered radio and became obsessed with looking at the careers of the people I admired, and I then started to think about how I could go about doing my own version of it.

One of the beautiful things about radio is that at its very best it is a companion for the listeners which can create a brilliantly mad community of people who all love hanging out together. I think the BBC is especially good at this as the only real agenda it has is making sure you have a nice time while listening. The BBC's three guiding principles are to 'educate, inform and entertain'. Translated into something that doesn't sound like it's in a sixth-form prospectus: 'tell people things that are true and do some fun shit'. That's it. There is a collective endeavour to the type of radio that I love and which keeps me interested to this day because you're allowed so much freedom to mess around with it. My favourite things: it's live, it's rooted in the day and, crucially, it's all about the listeners. The listeners are infinitely entertaining and funny. I also get immense joy from working in a big creative entity and I'd miss it greatly if I wasn't part of it. Radio 1 is powered by genius producers, expert music schedulers, talented journalists, some of the best engineers in the world, it has world-class marketing teams and a constant stream of brand-new, exciting presenters all hoping I die soon so the *Breakfast Show* is up for grabs again. Its whole is greater than the sum of its parts and it is a lovely club to be in. And to listen to. And I can say that confidently because I've listened to it for most of my life.

Conversely, one of the dangers of the way social media fame is set up and judged and therefore rewarded is that everything is about *you*. There is often no 'whole'. No team. No collaboration, no experienced producers to work with, no broadcaster to run the editorial checks by. It tends to be a solo endeavour and that's tough, exhausting and often lonely. And at its worst, it's horribly exposing because TikTok and Instagram tend to reward self-obsession. The satisfaction of creating something should always be the goal. And although in content creation that can be the case, it often gets diluted because while you can learn and fail and work out your niche, you don't have long. The money, notoriety and 'fame' might then come – but the *joy* was in the making (and the learning, and the failing). You need to be rubbish for a while in order to get really good before you're unleashed on the world. These sorts of careers, if you're serious about them, should be defined not by the quick buck or the one-off viral moment, but by longevity.

The focus a lot of the time seems to be in the hustle, in the flogging of a product, in the brand deal. But how long can that be sustained? Because take away the endorsement, and what have you actually made? You might have even had a community that believed in you, but you've sold them out. And who can blame you? The internet moves fast. So I'd always encourage young creatives to think smartly and use social media as a tool to market your well-thought-through funny ideas. Treat TikTok with the disdain with which it treats you. Use it as a shop window to show off how funny, smart and clever you are.

As brilliantly rewarding and far-reaching as social media is for creators, it's interesting to me that there is still a desire from many of them to transfer their skills into what you'd call more traditional mainstream media. Addison Rae is a good recent example. She started off putting herself through college by doing dances and small brand deals on TikTok but realised that she wanted to cement a more long-lasting legacy and has transitioned very cannily into an enormous pop star with a huge record deal with Sony. This is how new and old media can evolve together. Amelia Dimoldenberg is another brilliant example. Her Chicken Shop Date YouTube channel has served as an amazing audition for her to be given roles on television, radio and podcasts, and even to host on the red carpet at the Oscars and *Saturday Night Live*'s 50th birthday. She has ambitions to act and perform and no doubt she'll achieve them. And it all started online. That was her version of me doing hospital and community radio. She's been super smart in using her social media presence to ensure she doesn't just live in her own world but reaches the mainstream and has a career that lasts.

Just beware the traps, because you have to be ready for that big viral moment if it comes, and without the safety net of a manager or a producer or a boss, it could be really overwhelming and damaging. With all public-facing jobs where you're giving a part of yourself, you need support systems around you, good advice and people to make sure you're not being exploited. It can also be incredibly lonely. I've seen so many content creators talk about how they feel trapped by the niche content they make. You have to make sure you have a good load of people around you and if you do find online fame, you can all work on smart ways to diversify and make it last. Ten years ago, it would have been really damaging for me to dive headfirst into *Strictly*. I didn't do it because I didn't want to do it. But I only worked that out because I had really great professional advice around me. People that had seen it all before and could show me where the pitfalls were. It was a moment when I decided that if you join the circus, you can't take the piss out of it. I enjoy being a little bit out of the tent. Showbiz is weird and brutal so I've been careful to work out how much of it I want in my life.

I don't want to be disingenuous and pretend I don't like the attention. I love that some people love what I do; it makes it all worthwhile. I really *love* doing my job but it's still genuinely surprising when people say they listen to the show or one of my 8,000 podcasts. It'll be nice for there to be a new thing for people to mention to me when this book's out. So make sure you say nice things about it.

Of course one of the downsides of being known, and known for being friendly, is that you have to be on your best behaviour at all times. I do feel pressure to be nice the entire time even if I'm feeling tired and I'm in a dreadful mood. But 99 per cent of the time I love stopping and chatting to people, and I do think as someone in the public eye – who says every day how great the listeners are – it is part of my job. Because I do believe that. Living your values is important and it's the very least I can do. But it gets tested from time to time. Recently, my dad was quite seriously ill and spent a week in hospital with some very severe infections. Having to pretend that everything's fine and your dad's definitely not going to die is difficult, regardless of the job you're doing, but I'd say it's particularly weird if your job is one in which you have to perform and be fun at 7am. On one occasion, I was hurrying around the supermarket near the hospital getting supplies for my dad on the ward and a few bits for Mum to make sure she was looking after herself too when a really lovely woman stopped me by the mince to say how much the radio cheers her up in the morning. She told me that her mum had been ill recently and it was a lovely distraction every morning. Obviously that's absolutely amazing to hear, and yet I just wanted to scream and say, 'I'm so stressed and sad, my dad's next door on his deathbed please stop talking to me, I'm exhausted.' I didn't do that. Instead I gave her a few minutes of my time, asked after her mum who I don't know, said that the radio is a distraction for me when I'm feeling sad too, but I stopped short of telling her my worries because that would bring the mood down and I have to be happy when people meet me. You want to meet the radio me, right? Not the real, complex, human me. You want the 'singing the Animal News theme tune or doing an impression of the King shouting at his bagpiper out of the bedroom window' me! (It was reported a couple of years ago that the King has a bagpiper to wake him up at 9am every day.) And that's how it should be. Not the bagpiper, that's batshit, but the meeting me bit. Oh and the impression of King Prince Charles.

I don't want to bump into Michael Palin when he's not being lovely avuncular Michael Palin! Good customer service is important. My great friend and long-time radio producer Chris Sawyer's running joke if he's ever with me when I'm approached by people wanting to have a nice chat is that I fucked it when I decided to make 'being nice' one of my things. He's a cynical old hag and I remind him that I'm naturally pleasant and genuinely do like people and it isn't a persona. 'You'd have an easier life if you were a bit of a cunt,' he replies. Yeah, but I'd be a cunt. And that'd be awful. We agreed once that maybe being a 'comedy grump' would have been quite fun. There's still time for that, I guess. Maybe I'll be able to grow into more of a Larry David character as I age. That would be great fun. I love that grumpy old Jew so much. My idol. I read an interview with the actor Brian Cox and he apparently gets stopped by fans of the TV show *Succession* in which he played the cantankerous media mogul Logan Roy, and they request he tell them to 'FUCK OFFFFF!' in the style of his character. Maybe that gets just as tiring, but at least the bar is set at a place where he can be rude without ruining anyone's day. Quite the opposite.

I also am capable of being really grumpy but I feel like I absolutely cannot let it show (apart from in the chapter 'I'm Not Coming to Your Wedding in Greece'). Everyone (me included) *loves* hearing if someone well known has kicked off so I'm always aware that if someone is rude to me, jumps the queue I'm in, tries to run me over, has a go at me online, punches me, kidnaps my dog, has an affair with my wife or kills my nan (good luck with that one, she's already dead), I can't rise to it. I'm Mr Nice. I've been programmed not to react. Much like I did to my dog, we trained him to be less reactive using repetition and reward with real-life situations and a lot of squeezy cheese. I underwent a six-week residential course in 2007 where I ate half my bodyweight in Primula but my god am I good at keeping calm if I'm face-to-face with someone who wants a reaction from me. However, if I'm tired – which, let's face it, is often

– I might let myself down. Usually it's travel-related. I get annoyed at buses that drive too fast, for example. I can't stand it when people drive really close to me when I'm on my bike and that's my weakness. I get into full-blown slanging matches sometimes and I surprise myself with how quickly I become foul-mouthed and 'Bromley'. I've kicked a few vans, knocked on countless windows and gestured to a few surprised drivers. I think it stems from a) feeling incredibly vulnerable next to a big hulking lorry and b) thinking about how embarrassing it would be for my life to end on my shitty little bike at the hands of some moron in a gilet driving a Tesla who was on his phone and not concentrating. Disclaimer: most drivers are very tolerant of us annoying cyclists but also, I get it! I'm not always included in 'us cyclists' and when I'm driving and a cyclist is behaving like a dick, I'll get *so* annoyed with them. The duality of man.

I also hate jobsworths in airports, train stations, customer services, how slow HMRC are at rebates even though they'll fine you if your tax return is a day late (fuck you!), EDF Energy, Thames Water and one of the pubs near Radio 1 that appears to hate customers. Or maybe just me. Basically anyone in these roles that deliberately goes out of their way to make things more difficult for you should proceed immediately to the bin. But obviously I can't ever say what I really want to because it might be filmed and go viral.

This happened to me a couple of years ago. There was a TikTok that gained a lot of traction from a bloke who said that I was his 'nemesis'. I kept getting tagged in it and I was genuinely excited to watch it because it's a funny idea to have a comedy 'nemesis'. Personally, I've got loads. I don't really wish them ill but it's funny to have a pantomime villain or two in your life. I class anyone who does a show on commercial radio as one of mine, for instance. Anyway, as I started to watch this video, I quickly realised that he was entirely humourless about the whole thing and told a really boring story about me jumping the queue in Starbucks once upon a time and it was less about a silly celeb story and more about the fact he clearly hated my guts. I had and still have no recollection of jumping the queue but on the radio I made as much of a joke as I could about it. That's the thing – you have to try to laugh these things off because otherwise they can escalate and you'll look humourless. I wanted to tell him to piss off and get a fucking life for trying to smear my name, but sadly that isn't allowed at that time of day and would have probably made things worse. If I saw him again in Starbucks, or any shop for that matter, I'd push in again, by the way. I'm nice most of the time but I can be incredibly petty. And he's clearly a twat.

Nemesis
Inferno

While I'm riled up and on the subject of people that annoy you, let's do a list. When you're a kid, you quite often have a series of enemies. A teacher maybe, a sibling, the kid at school who laughed at your sunglasses once and you still hate him for it. The important thing about having a nemesis is that they don't know they are your nemesis. They get to go through life blissfully unencumbered by the knowledge that you hate their guts. It's very teenage. Your hormones are out of control but in the spirit of 'don't lose sight of your younger self', who said all those things have to be positive?! Here I am a grown man, very busy, very grateful and yet I still find I have plenty of time to hate certain things and people. I think it's healthy. I'm only friends with people who are able to say something devastating about someone else. It's unnatural to like everyone and everything.

So, without further ado, here's my list of nemeses:

* The aforementioned radio presenters.
* Wind.
* Birds flapping their wings near me.
* People who make being left-handed their entire personality (Bella does this).

* Business podcasts – or any podcasts, but oddly usually business ones, where the aim is to get the guests to cry, or the listeners to buy their stupid supplements.
* Money giveaways on commercial radio (they're just fleecing the listeners because it costs three quid to enter and that's what makes the prize fund – don't be fooled).
* The Nissan Qashqai.
* People with private jets.
* Dubai.
* Any TikTok account that stops people in the street for content (it's an immediate block).
* People who say holibobs.
* People who do the 'face for radio' joke.
* Paddington (the bear, and the station at the weekend).
* The phrase 'wherever you get your podcasts'.
* Alan Sugar.
* Our elderly neighbour, who I spotted protesting outside an abortion clinic.
* Skrillex.
* Marios (Bella's ex-boyfriend who was an ultimate fighter. Apparently he's lovely. I don't give a shit.).
* People who aren't farmers that wear gilets.
* The guy that leaves bread out for the foxes on our street every night.
* Channel 4 after they cancelled my TV show *Rise and Fall*.
* Any cricket podcast that I don't present.
* People who make their dog their entire personality (yes, you can be your own nemesis).

All the best for the future

* Huel and anyone who drinks/flogs it.
* Mummy and Daddy bloggers (maybe not all of them. Hmmm. No, actually, all of them. I just find it uncomfortable that the kids in question have had no say in whether they want their entire childhood broadcast to millions of people. How damaging might that be?! Also, commodifying your kid to get freebies is totally end-of-days dystopian batshit.)

Daddy Issues

On the subject of kids, here's the chapter we've all been waiting for, the reason we've all been put on this earth ... to procreate! I don't know if that's true, though, because no one knows why we're here and everyone's definition of the Meaning of Life is different.

I always thought I'd have kids and I think I wanted them but only because I didn't employ any critical thought. It just felt like something you would automatically do, and for hundreds of millions of people that is exactly how it goes. As I mentioned earlier, you can go through the *Mario Kart* checkpoints: get a job, get married, buy a house, have kids, go bald, get cancer, die. And that's great, by the way. Well, not the cancer bit but as long as the rest of it is what you definitely want, well done you. The thing that baffles me to this day is that not one person along the way told me I had a choice in the matter. Nobody said, 'You know what, you don't have to have children and you could still have a nice fulfilling life.' Certainly no one mentioned how hard it might be to have them in the first place. It was just expected that I'd grow up, find a birthing partner and make new humans. It seems like it's the default accepted path for all of us and that's mad. It's too big a decision to not give careful consideration to and I genuinely think people give more thought to researching the spec on a new car than they do to starting a family. 'Alloy wheels, metallic paint, cruise control is useful on the motorway and yeah, we'll probably have a couple of kids I guess.'

Having children is an enormous decision to make. It's also an enormous privilege to even be physically *able* to have them. Starting a family is utterly life-changing in brilliant ways (so I've been told) and also sometimes in horrendous ways (so I've also been told – *a lot*). And it's a decision not to be taken lightly and certainly not something to sleepwalk into. If you're not sure whether you want to have kids, I'd say it's better to not bother because no one wants a half-arsed parent. No one could ever accuse my mum and dad of being that and as Bella pointed out very early on in our relationship, they think the sun shines out of my arse (they're right). Bella and I, over the years, have had endless chats about whether to have kids or not and I've been encouraged to think much more deeply about it all as I've gone from my early thirties to my late thirties.

I began to think about what my parents' lives would have been like if they hadn't had kids, and who's to say they wouldn't have had just as good a time as they have, albeit in a completely different way? Without me and my sister, my mum wouldn't have had to stop teaching for long periods of time, that's for sure. Undoubtedly, having us made promotions and new opportunities much harder to go for. Similarly, my dad almost worked himself into an early grave to earn enough money in incredibly stressful roles at some very challenging schools to provide for the family. There was a period of my early teens where I barely saw him because the job was all-consuming and he'd have felt tremendous pain about not being more present. And Dad, obviously you're reading this – you still managed to be completely amazing at it and I feel so lucky to say that you still are. In fact, we're currently on a weekend away together and I'm sitting here writing while he's sitting next to me watching *The Day of the Jackal* with a red wine in his hand (he loves assassins). Barney's here too and he's currently licking his very small penis. His penis, not my dad's, I should clarify.

My mum and dad don't (to my knowledge) have any regrets about having children but the fact remains that with two fewer people in the family, they would both have been able to work on themselves more. They would have been able to enjoy each other in different ways and seen each other more as adults and less as 'mum' and 'dad', but one of their dreams was to have children and they would tell you they've loved devoting a vast portion of their lives to us. I can't express how grateful I am for that. All I'm putting across is that I don't feel the same urge to do that and I think that's OK. I don't want to give up the dynamic that Bella and I (plus Barney) have managed to build. Life gets busy and even without children, I don't feel as though I see as much of her or Barney as I want to. I don't want to add a child into this and end up being able to hang out with them even less. After all, I fell in love with her because of who she is and who we are together, not because I thought she'd be a great vessel for a baby. This isn't to say that I hate children or hate people that have children (apart from the aforementioned influencers that monetise their poor offspring before they're old enough to have a choice in the matter). I completely understand the appeal if it's right for you. In fact, I'm envious of people that are certain about wanting them because that's wonderful clarity of thought and much like most of my friends that have had or are having that urge, I'm incredibly happy for them. I'll be there helping out when I can. Listening to you moan. Entertaining you when you get a night off and hanging out with your kids as wacky Uncle Greg until we both get bored and I can hand them back with an enormous sigh of relief.

I'm lucky that I have so many great kids in my life. My sister was the first to have them, back in 2008 when Pia was born. I'd just started out at Radio 1 and she was the first baby I'd really ever hung out with and I couldn't believe how fun it was to be an uncle. It still is, even though Pia, my niece, and Tom, my nephew, are now teenagers and amazingly uninterested in almost everything I can offer. Apart from tickets to see Billie Eilish, cheeky gits. I'm so glad I had a sibling to give me the opportunity to have nieces and nephews. My sister is the most extraordinary person – she's the best. She went through many of the life checkpoints before I did and I watched on in awe as she became a monstrous teenager, then went off to university (Cambridge – she's the smart one), brought boyfriends home, got a cool job, earned decent money, bought her first flat all off her own back, fell in love, had kids and got married. She's amazing and because of the age gap, I've always felt like I had two mums. The ten years between us often raises a few eyebrows when I tell people and the reason is very in keeping with this chapter so it feels appropriate to share. My parents had great difficulty in conceiving and that period of their lives, they've since told me, was full of incredibly upsetting events. They lost a child and that's something you never get over. Never query why there's a big age gap between siblings unless it naturally comes up in conversation. At the very least you're being nosy but at worst, the reason could be incredibly sad and traumatic. In fact, don't ever be a fucking busybody and ask questions prying into whether someone is having kids – questions like that are best avoided. We should try to resist having an opinion on when, why and how people have babies. There isn't a perfect age gap, you don't need an explanation as to why people don't or can't have them and really we should all keep our noses out because we don't know what's going on with people. It's incredibly private and none of anyone's business. It might be a choice or it might be a private struggle. AVOID.

Having children is one option but it isn't the only one. We have way more choice in our lives than we realise and shouldn't feel pressured by anyone into doing anything just because we think that's just what you do or should do. I didn't realise until a couple of years ago that life would be OK without having children. Having a family still seems to be the done thing and maybe it'll be wonderful for you, but I'm here to remind you that you could just as happily skip through life prioritising your partner, your dog, your hobbies, your community, your nieces and nephews, your friends' smelly children and perhaps most importantly, yourself. And it can all be fun.

It's estimated that one in eight pregnancies ends in miscarriage, which makes them very common, but despite this they're really not talked about enough and they really should be because the whole thing is incredibly traumatic. Bella miscarried a few years ago after conceiving accidentally and we felt fucking embarrassed about it, particularly as we hadn't decided to actively try. We, like many couples, were in the 'Oh yeah, maybe it'll be fun' stage of the decision-making process and hadn't thought it through properly. I refer you to my earlier point: if you're not sure you want to go through with it – don't. Or at least give the decision the reverence it deserves. This isn't to be taken lightly, and yet some people do. We did! And even though the entire grisly, upsetting process of going through a miscarriage is enough to make you never want to have sex again, the episode shocked us into thinking properly about it all. Not just 'Do I want to put my wife through that again?' but on a larger scale, 'Do we want to have another person in our lives forever?'

I'm convinced that lots of people only really think about having a 'baby' and they don't consider that one day they will no longer have a baby but instead an annoying 14-year-old. Reminder: they GROW UP! And they're there all the time. It's not just a few years of a cute little thing you can exploit for likes on Instagram. Get a dog if you want to do that. Little humans stick around and dominate your entire life. A few questions to consider: Do you want your life to fundamentally change? Can you afford it? Can you fit them in your flat? Are you willing to give up lots and lots of time? Do you want to drive them to swimming every Tuesday? Do you want to take them on every holiday you go on? Wake up early every time you have a day off because kids never have a day off being a kid? Do you want to look after someone every day for 18 years only for them to think that you're the lamest, oldest, most boring person in the world and then after draining you of all your energy and money they go off and make their own way in the world, no longer needing you? Are you ready to worry constantly that your entire personality is now 'mum' or 'dad' and become unsure of who you even are anymore? That final question came from a friend of mine who's got kids, took a look at this paragraph and wanted me to add it in. Yikes.

Bella and I took the discussion to a deliberately silly conclusion but we answered the essential question of 'Do you want your current life and relationship with each other to fundamentally change forever?' with a resounding 'no'. And that's fine. If that all sounds great and you think I'm being over dramatic and you love the sound of all that (because I also get that lots of it would be great fun), then that's brilliant for you. I'm just being silly for a funny-ish book. But mine and Bella's truth is in there somewhere. Another great fear that people have is the idea that you'll get old and regret not having them. The most common age to have children for women in the UK is 30. That was ages ago for us. I'm 39 and Bella is 41 – quite old in terms of baby-making. I might be wrong but I feel like I would have felt the regret set in by now. I've lived a lot of my life without them so far and it's not felt like there was anything missing. We've seen so many babies come into the world and not one of them has made us go, 'Oh yeah, we should have one.'

Get
a Dog
Instead

Perhaps the regret is being staved off by having a very demanding dog instead. Despite knowing what dogs were from a very early age, they just weren't part of my childhood. I didn't even bother badgering my parents for one because obviously they'd have been the ones that ended up looking after it and they were too busy working for that. In that situation, it's a well-trodden path that stressed parents de-escalate the situation by opting for either a fish or some sort of rodent. Usually a hamster. We were very much a Hamster House™. But here we are, I'm now a full-blown dog guy. I never thought I'd be a dog person. And yet I am. Unbearably so. Barney is at least 65 per cent of my personality and 85 per cent of my social media game. It's got to be better than making your job your personality though, eh? Having a dog, and read these words carefully, is a complete fucking nightmare. Honestly. I can't believe that there's an ACTUAL ANIMAL in my house: a weird creature that can't talk and is just living with us as if it is the most normal thing. He farts all the time, leaves hair everywhere, barks anytime there's a noise outside or if I don't pay him enough attention, wakes me up early by hitting me over the head with his paw at the weekend because he needs to have a wee, churns the grass up every time he goes out into the garden, traipses mud through the house, can't be left alone for more than three or four hours, needs hours of walks a day and is the main topic of conversation between Bella and me.

I've just come back from a walk with Barney and as I was bending down to pick up his latest deposit, the bag turned inside out on my hand, blowing in the wind and doubling back over the hot present before I could gather it all. The streetlight was behind me, my body casting a shadow, and I had to pull out my phone and shine the torch on the ground in order to see the remains I still needed to scoop up. Barney, who had done his business, was keen to keep walking so I was crouching down while being pulled away as the wind picked up. Out loud I said, 'What the fuck is happening here?!'

Why did we choose this? It's a good question.

I don't know. But what I do know is that I'm completely obsessed with him, I can't believe how much I love him and I wouldn't change a single thing about him, apart from maybe the farts. They really are heinous. He cleared a dinner party once because they were so bad. Someone genuinely went home. He is also hilarious. I belly laugh at the things he does every single day. His stupid little face. The way he sleeps on his back with all four legs in the air. I think about him all the time, especially if I'm doing something I don't want to be – *What's Barney doing?* I wonder. I'd just rather be at home with him following me around the house hoping I'll give him some cheese. I'm more fond of him than I am of lots of humans I've met. He's one of my best friends. And that will sound absolutely insane to many of you.

It would have sounded mad to me a few years ago. In fact, before Barney, I remember someone at work taking a couple of days off when their dog died and I thought it was 'a bit much'.

I'm deeply embarrassed by that reaction now because a) it's unkind and b) I would do the same now. I'd have to take a couple of months off. Ours is a bond I just didn't understand and now I can't remember my life without him. Despite him being an absolute maniac, we got really lucky with Barney. He's an amazingly gentle soul, anxious as hell but so sweet. I remember the moment we met for the first time at Battersea Dogs & Cats Home in 2019 so vividly. This eight-month-old gangly little thing bounded up to me and jumped up to say hello. It was honestly love at first sight. Bella even took a photo of the moment (and then subsequently put that photo on a T-shirt for me, which I wear regularly). We nervously took him home a couple of days later in a cab and it was completely terrifying. Neither of us knew what we'd done. Bella wanted a nice ageing little dog (in her head it was called Mary) and here I was forcing an enormous, big-pawed labrador puppy into our lives.

My god the first few months were hard. Countless big shits on the floor when I came downstairs in the morning, most of our shoes were eaten, several charger cables were chewed through, the *actual wall* was chomped into at one point. I had a truly horrible dark thought once after I was mopping up yet another 5am runny puddle of horror that if I accidentally left the front door open then he might just leave and never come back and it wouldn't technically be my fault. That's a bad one, isn't it? Even today on the walk he was a complete nightmare. He's got a new habit of taking me to Pets at Home whenever we do a road walk and although it's slightly tedious, I have no choice but to find it adorable as he is very much in charge, locking his legs up if I try to take him in another direction. I get it, though. If I was him, I'd want to go to Pets at Home every day because it's unlimited food, unlimited toys and unlimited treats in a pick-and-mix-style dispenser. All the staff fuss over him as soon as he ambles in. It's heaven. He knows what he likes, he knows what brings him joy. He's very in touch with prioritising pleasure. That's his reason for being.

Between March 2020 and March 2021, 3.2 million households added a pet to their family. That's an extraordinary number and there are now 12 million dogs in the UK so they must be doing something right. Conversely, worldwide, there is a decline in human birth rates. There are more people deciding not to have children (or to have fewer) than previous generations. This is undoubtedly interesting to me, so why are we so obsessed with our pets? Our lives are already stressful and yet we think a dog will solve everything. But in my limited experience so far, they sort of do. For all his idiocy, his mania, his energy and his foul smells, Barney doesn't stop the stresses of my life from arriving but he does give me a break from them all. A break from all the chatter and noise, the news, the world and the associated brain clutter. A break from humans. Maybe that's it. He's not going to let me down by cancelling on me, he's not going to break my heart by falling in love with someone else, he's not going to bitch about me behind my back or steal any of my things. He's fiercely loyal, he depends on me to keep him alive and as long as I do that, in return he gives me so much joy, so much oxytocin when we roll around together and SO much viral content. But more than all of that, he takes me out of myself and returns me to an even keel if I get too high on my own fumes or too low on the toxic ones the world can pump out. He teaches me how to be a good dog owner and he offers a constant reminder to check my selfishness levels. And he does all of this without uttering a word. Come to think of it, dogs might just be magic. So, yeah, if you want to be cute about it, you could say we chose dogs instead of kids, but that's doing both a disservice. It's not an either/or. Or a question of having a kid or a dog! Do what you want. There's no one right answer, much like there's no right way about doing life. Except when it comes to cats. Cats can fuck off.

Are We Nearly There Yet?

Almost from the moment you're born, there's a lot of pressure to excel at everything, it comes at you from all sides. So much pressure is put on *firsts*. The first word, the first step, the first time you did a sick on your dad. Not to mention the first time you write down a word or manage to put a triangle block into a triangle hole. 'SHE'S A GENIUS!' Equally, I know many parents that worry their child has fallen behind somehow. For example, just because your kid repeatedly takes a stool over to the sofa and tries to sit on it while wobbling on the soft unstable cushions, resulting in him falling off repeatedly, doesn't mean he's going to grow up stupid. This may or may not have happened to Bella's nephew this morning.

What's that annoying saying? 'Life comes at you fast!' It's true, though; just a few short years after we're out of the womb we're thrown into a system which ranks us from smartest to thickest, and that's before we even reach school. Who's got the highest reading age? Who's got the neatest handwriting? Who didn't piss themselves in the reading area? Obviously, I know that reading and writing are incredibly important. And so is learning how to count, even if you do have a calculator everywhere you go in the form of your phone these days. But you're not more of a person if you don't excel in the formal ways that a school tracks. Perhaps you have other interests in the world, perhaps your brain just learns differently. No two brains are the same and thankfully the world is slowly waking up to this. Neurodivergent conditions and disorders are being taken far more seriously in schools and workplaces than they were even a few years ago, and this is great progress. There's a lot to undo, though, and these antiquated structures take time to remodel. We'll get there. But for now, kids will have to make do with the terror of the exam room. If you fail an exam, are you toast? If you pass an exam, are you a legend? No, not really. Yes, you might either be proud or disappointed but it won't be the making or indeed the breaking of you. And yet everyone's obsessed with tests. You can pass zero exams or 300 and it won't determine whether or not you have a shit life. They are an unavoidable part of the society we live in, so all you can do is try your best, take what you can from them and then work out what to do when they're done and dusted – but no one is better or worse for having taken exams.

The tricky thing about spending as many as 21 years operating within this highly tested, competitively ranked system is that you run the risk of seeing everything else you do in life through this lens. This mentality can show itself by wanting the best car or house on the street, the most well-paid job or even, most dispiritingly, feeling the nagging need to be brilliant at the things you do in your spare time. You don't have to compete in every aspect of your life just because they made us sit exams as teenagers. You don't always have to excel. There is still joy to be found in being completely shit at something you love, but it's easy to forget because the culture we live in strongly implies you have to be constantly striving to be the best, beat everyone, be the richest, be the most successful – in all categories. But you don't have to be amazing at everything. Or indeed anything!

Maybe there's some wisdom in the old saying 'it's the journey not the destination'? No one's checking in on whether you are any good at the interests you have. These things are for you to take whatever you want out of them. There are hobbies and sports that I constantly wrestle with and give up on because I don't think I'm good enough at them. I absolutely love playing the piano, for example, but I'm annoyed I'm not very good at it so I don't bother doing it much. Instead I end up mindlessly sitting on my phone looking at dashcam footage of car crashes. That's a real shame. And also quite odd. I also stopped doing art at school because I got terrible grades, but spending time drawing something or using paints to make a huge mess on a bit of paper is a brilliant thing to do to calm my brain. I lose confidence because I think I should be as good as Monet. (*Heyyyy, I must be the Monet!* I think to myself. You should listen to the audiobook because written down here that joke doesn't work nearly as well.)

Maybe this book should have been called *Chill the Fuck Out*. Because that's what I'd have loved someone to tell me when I was getting obsessed with not being the best cricketer in the team/ club/county/world when I was a teenager. I forgot to enjoy it. I forgot to have fun. I was too stressed about getting out and what that would mean. If I wasn't going to compete profession-ally, what was the point? That attitude meant I completely forgot about why I loved the game in the first place.

When was the last time you did something just for the sake of doing it and not because you thought you'd be good at it? I don't want this to turn into an overt self-help book but those things are *really* great for your brain. Do more things you're shit at, it's liberating. I'm not very good at gardening but I absolutely love getting out there and pretending I know what I'm doing. I'm a very good clearer, a good trimmer and a good mower, but aside from that, I haven't a clue. I'll plant stuff confidently and then realise two weeks later it's not working so I'll dig it up and put it somewhere else – no one's marking me on it. I don't need to be an award-winning gardener; I don't even really want to get much better at it, and that makes me very happy. I like being puzzled by plants. You don't have to understand everything.

Yoga is another thing that I'm dreadful at but I've been doing it online with a teacher called Nat for a few years now and it absolutely saved me in the pandemic because it gave me something else to focus on. I am tall, I am limby and my god do I look stupid doing a cat cow but does it give me joy? Huge amounts. Yes, I've got a bit better over the years but I haven't become obsessed with it. In fact (and sorry if you're reading this, Nat), I sort of dread it. But I force myself to do it because I always feel better afterwards and it's good to stop my brain whirring for an hour. It has made me calmer, it's made my body more flexible, I'm better at running because my muscles don't seize up anymore but do I want to learn more about it and master it? No. Absolutely not. I've been doing roughly the same moves for three years and I love it. So why change it? It's for *me*, and no one else. I also joined an expensive gym at the start of last year and, on the whole, I love it and it's changed my life. I'm not doing anything groundbreaking but along with some small tweaks to my diet (less sugar, cutting down on white bread and no heavy red meat), I just do stuff to build my strength. I feel approximately 1,000 times better than I did 18 months ago. I'm not going because I want to get a six-pack or to wow everyone with the gun show but I've leaned up and I feel stronger, more energetic and … dare I say it … younger. The eagle-eyed among you will have noticed that I said 'on the whole, I love it'. That's because it's a gym often frequented by actors. Famously the most aesthetically gifted people on the planet. They sometimes have to do six-week bursts of mega training to get ready for a role which, although it's a great way to dispel the myths of Hollywood (it's part of their job to look unnaturally ripped), it's undeniably devastating to walk into the induction day and have to work out next to celebrated movie hunk Leo Woodall looking like the love child of Adonis and Aphrodite. He's 'THE BOY' in that final Bridget Jones – *Mad About the Boy* – for fuck's sake. First world problems, I realise.

For Christmas last year, Bella bought me, the boy *she's* mad about, an Airfix kit. I'd never bothered with Airfix as a kid, and after spending ten days making a small-scale model of an old naval helicopter called a Sea King, I remembered why. The idea of having to make your own toy before you get to play with it seemed truly insane to me when I was growing up. I had a huge interest in remote-controlled cars, model aeroplanes, Scalextric, miniature railways … all the good stuff, but I could never get my head around why you'd want to spend hours glueing it all together before you got to play with it. I wanted to have my fun there and then. Done. Finished. Ready to be used. I don't think that's an unusual reaction either; impatience is built into many of us and arguably attention spans are getting worse. I do think I'm making progress with my patience as I get older. I mean, writing a book takes patience in itself. That said, I can't wait for this book to be published, sell a million copies and maybe even win the Best Book of All Time award, and sometimes I wish it was just done so I could enjoy pretentiously telling everyone about 'the writing process' and how 'most of it was done in the bath' (that's true by the way). But as my nose hairs grow and my eyesight worsens, I understand more than ever that the end result is always made better by the joy you took from the process. In writing this I'm learning new things about myself, enjoying reminiscing about the old days and also surprising myself when I write something I find genuinely funny. It'll feel so much better on publication day when I know how long I spent on this. Lots of people get their books written for them because they think 'doing a book' is more important than 'writing a book'. Easy come, easy go, as they say. I don't know who 'they' are, but it's largely true in life. It's a trap we can all fall into, and not just when writing a book or dealing with a model kit.

The model I sweated over for hours is passable and I'm certainly no pro (some might say the same about this book, although they'd be wrong, of course) but the point is ... I did it! And I didn't think of anything else while I was doing it. The noise of the world was muted and the helicopter became my sole focus. I was peaceful, for the most part: there were a handful of times I wanted to hurl it at the wall, but only a handful and I managed not to. On the finished product – which is proudly displayed near the TV – there are scuffed paint marks and parts that wobble, and even after all that work, it doesn't *do* anything. And that's fine. The entire joy of the kit turned out to come from the (often) quite frustrating process. A metaphor for life, maybe. As is what happened at Christmas when my brilliant friend Jenny was dancing in the living room at my house after 300 glasses of wine and knocked it off the shelf while pirouetting, breaking it in two, proving yet again how common helicopter crashes are. She's devastated about this and will hate that it's made the book. Hi Jenny; you're forgiven. Love you x

Brain Rot

The Airfix was a sweet relief from being constantly attached to a phone that demands I look at it once every two minutes at least. When I'm really tired, I constantly and moronically flick between apps, desperately trying to avoid boredom. At least I think that's what it is. It might also be fear of missing out on something, or attempting to find something that stops me from having to engage my brain to try to tackle the 1,000 things I should be doing. It's a comfort blanket that rarely provides comfort and tends to instead provide numbness. A numbness blanket. As I scroll, I feel my brain rotting sometimes but I just can't stop checking, clicking, swiping and liking. After a good session of watching the world flash past my eyes, the devastating thing is, I very rarely actually like anything I've just seen – let alone remember it.

The internet is the most incredible thing that's happened in our lifetime and it's changed the world, simultaneously bringing everyone closer together and pushing us further apart – and sometimes making us all feel unbearably alone. My phone offers access to every brilliant person in my life and yet I spend most of my time watching old cricket highlights or, worse, fucking idiots driving through flood water. At the time of writing, I'm also getting a lot of Paul Mescal videos, which isn't a bad thing – he's a nice man and looks GREAT in short shorts – but I know too much about him at this point.

I wonder if we're getting more comfortable not seeing our friends, or is that just a consequence of getting older and busier? Maybe it's both. But just look around you now, if you're out in public, and you'll see most people alone, staring down at their phones, not engaging with the world around them. Not even looking up when walking because they're convinced what's in the palm of their hand at that moment is the most important thing in the world. Of course, the chances are, it won't be. It'll be a video of Moo Deng the pygmy hippo or someone boring oversharing on a podcast and crying. WHY ARE YOU TELLING US THIS! The other problem is that it's just too much information for us to deal with. It's both amazing and distressing in equal measure that we can search for anything instantly and find the answer to any question in a matter of seconds. For example, I tried a few very random questions to see what I could find:

What is the loudest fart ever recorded?

On 11 May 1972, Paul Hunn farted for a staggering 2 minutes and 42 seconds. It was recorded at 118.1 decibels. Good going, Paul.

What school did Hitler go to?

Adolf Hitler went to Volksschule primary school in Fischlham. Eh, now you know.

What car does the presenter Adrian Chiles drive?

This was the hardest of all the questions. He's elusive is our Adrian, but after a couple of minutes, I found an article where it seems he owned a fairly run-of-the-mill BMW 5 Series. Diesel.

All the best for the future

Even when we aren't endlessly scrolling social media there are WhatsApp groups popping off all day long, but how much of that is meaningful and stimulating conversation and how much of it is just memes and Alan Partridge quotes? The simple answer is that both objectives can be achieved. You can be healthily obsessed with your phone, be chronically online and love some of the fun, information and connectivity it gives you, as long as you realise this can't be *instead* of actual face-to-face human interaction. It's tempting to think you've caught up with a friend by sending them a video of a dog smiling, and while this is definitely a lovely thing to do – I do it *all* the time – you do also have to follow it up at some point with a meaningful act of in-person friendship. Memes and things are good at keeping the friendship simmering but we were put on earth to interact physically so let's make sure we do – otherwise, our friendships will become parasocial and you might as well be best mates with a computer.

Phones aren't all bad though, of course. I get exhausted with the 'you're always on your phone' brigade because YES! Of course I am! Everyone I've ever met, all the funniest people in the world, my job, my money, my fun, every song ever recorded, my favourite memes and all the books ever written are on this thing I can hold in my hand! Why wouldn't I be on it a lot? I'm guilty of being on my phone too much but that's because I get a lot out of it. My career has been massively boosted because I've always been interested in making little bits of content. I love making stupid videos, trying out jokes and 'bits' on social media and I have to be on top of current pop culture stuff – a lot of which will end up on the radio. It's a great place to try stuff out and work out what people like. It can be a very useful creative outlet, and it connects me with such a great audience and obviously I'm going to flog the fuck out of this book on there, so I'm eternally grateful for and proud of the following of weirdos that I've amassed over the years. I love the communities that can be created online; it's everything I wanted as a kid but better, because then I had to settle for AOL forums and MSN Messenger. Kids now would look at the Nokia 3210 and think it came from 1810. That said, there are certainly times when I look back at that time (not 1810, I mean my childhood) with a wistful nostalgia. We've lost the balance. If we didn't make a conscious effort, we genuinely wouldn't need to leave the house for weeks on end. Everything you could need can be brought to the door, all the entertainment can be streamed into our living rooms, all our friends are there at the touch and swipe of a screen.

I *do* worry about being a moron, though, and I try to catch myself mindlessly scrolling because it does nothing for me. A little scroll here and there can sometimes find some gold. Radio wise, I've found so many great things over the years doing that and being chronically online. Britain's tallest duck, Long Boi, was sent to me on Instagram, I started chatting to Francis Bourgeois on TikTok, I discovered Djo's music on there too. In fact, the painting of the guy from the nineteenth century that looks quite a lot like me was sent to me by countless listeners via social media a few years ago. It's now on the back cover of this book (go on, look) and, alongside me on a wrecking ball, is one of the most searched things about me.

All that is fine and fun but when your brain's gone into safe mode and you're not even taking it in, STOP. It's so weird. I'm going to have a little scroll now and report back what comes up and let's see if any of it's useful:

A load of students trying to stop a bus sliding down the hill in the snow. Quite funny.

SWIPE.

A weird video of a cartoon wasp playing the guitar.

SWIPE.

A clip of a podcast about spies. Looks shit.

SWIPE.

A clip from a parenting podcast. Looks even shitter.

SWIPE.

Dashcam of a girl being pulled over by the police on her driving test. Not as fun as I'd hoped.

SWIPE.

Olivia Colman reading a *CBeebies Bedtime Story*. Really great. That is good.

SWIPE.

A guy dropping an entire tray full of glasses of white wine. The pick of the bunch. Excellent.

What has that done for my day? Well, on this occasion it's added a hundred words to the count of this book but it's done nothing to enhance my life or my brain. I've tried to get into the habit of going towards a news or sports app or just starting up a podcast episode instead of scrolling social media when I'm feeling restless and often that works for me. It's good to fight back a bit with some broccoli when everyone's offering you pizza and ice cream.

Social media promised to connect us to the world, help us stay in touch with friends and bring us closer together. Sure, there's a bit of that, but for the most part all it's done is erase nuanced discussion to the point where people just hurl insults at each other, encourage people to mine the depths of their souls publicly in order to cut through and gain attention, push us towards displaying a perfect-looking life in order to make everyone feel like they're missing out on something, and make Andrew Tate famous. Well done, everyone! Smashed it.

I have made some great online friends over the years and I promise to meet them in real life for a beer at some point. My wife actually started off as an online friend on Twitter – which is now of course a complete fucking garbage fire. I did well to use it as a dating app, actually. If I was looking for a partner on Twitter now, I wouldn't have found the insanely talented, funny and beautiful Bella Mackie but instead I fear I'd have ended up marrying a radicalised racist called Wyatt who lives in Arkansas and has formed a questionably close relationship with the goat he met on the long walk back from the annual demolition derby in 2017. Hey, look, who am I to judge? Wyatt, the goat and I could be living a very happy life on his ranch. I bet I'd be using my phone less – the signal would be bad and Wyatt would probably restrict the amount of contact I'd be allowed to have with the outside world, plus he'd no doubt believe that 5G would give me cancer and allow Bill Gates to spy on us. No, I can see it!

I'd turn into his sexy Ranch Wife, cooking up delicious mince-and-cheese-based dishes ready for when he returns home after an exhausting day hauling cattle. Perhaps Wyatt's offering me a better life?! Bella doesn't even let me have meat in the house. I'm not ashamed to say that I just googled 'Ranch Wife' to see if it was an actual thing and it is! Here comes another online rabbit hole to fall down.

It's odd that everyone feels like they have to perform for the camera constantly. No good deed goes un-posted, no family birthday unmined for likes. It's the bit of my job that can feel the most exhausting and intrusive but it *is* part of my job because I want people to get a sense of who I am. It's weird that everyone feels like they have to do it, though. You really don't have to! Maybe the worst part of the internet is the pressure to perform and engage. Unless it's paying you and therefore part of your career, why would you sell off parts of your actual life for no gain? The hack here might be to stop adding to the mess unless we absolutely have to and instead channel our energy into our real lives and real friends. Come to think of it, there's a real jumble of purposes on social media isn't there. Contained within your phone is all recorded music, constant updates from the world's celebrities, breaking news from every corner of the globe as well as your mate Sophie's hen-do in Brighton, and the photos from your holiday in Bali. Everything's content! And it's all competing with each other all of the time. The way we've been trained by these social media companies to ensure we're addicted helps reinforce the idea that every life event is another milestone to reach or checkpoint to go through. A huge part of the planning of an engagement announcement, for example, now appears to be making sure there's an accompanying social media strategy and roll-out plan. This is endemic through the celebrity/influencer world. How many collaboration posts have you seen from well-known couples telling you they're about to have another child? I know it might be part of their brand but it's an incredibly private, personal moment in their lives – is making it into content healthy? I don't know. It's even more bizarre and creepy to me that non-famous couples act as if there's a social media strategy behind their announcements too. I think we might look back at this period in a few years' time and think that some of this posting to get likes and attention was a bit reckless.

We could all do with looking at how reliant we are on our phones, but there's no need to beat ourselves up about it all; we're all savvy digital natives and that can open up amazing possibilities and opportunities, so it's not always a waste of time. Why is sitting on your phone any different from some of the stuff the old farts that moan about us doing that did in their youth? They used to sit around playing with a hoop and a stick or reading the newspaper. It just looked classier than staring at your hand. I wouldn't want to live in the old days; I love how immediate things can be. I love the communities you can join that make you feel less alone. How great is it that generations of teenagers are able to find allies going through the exact same things they are? I love that I can FaceTime my family wherever I am, I love that WhatsApp chats with friends can cheer me up instantly. Yes, of course, those things come with downsides but that is literally life. You can't have good without bad, light without dark and as I say regularly to my boss at Radio 1, you can't have a hit without a miss. He's unsure about this as an excuse for a bad feature.

Either way, I think it's a case of catching the madness before it sets in and trying not to kid ourselves that we're going to change our ways, buy a dumb phone and go cold turkey, never going on TikTok again — because that's just not true. Much like everything in our adult lives, we have to try hard to not be passive and stay alert to the tricks and traps that lurk.

Well done to you for managing to stay away from yours long enough to be able to concentrate on reading. You're engaging in a book instead of infecting your brain with moronic internet things! That's an achievement in itself. As a reward, go and watch some videos of things being squashed by a big metal crusher.

Don't Grow Up, It's a Trap

In general, you can tell someone's age by what their favourite social media platform is. Sure, this is somewhat reductive and sort of against my rule of 'people are many things' but it's also fun, therefore it fits the brief of the book – so up yours! It goes as follows:

* Kids: Snapchat.
* Teenagers: Snapchat, TikTok and maybe a bit of Instagram when they're allowed.
* Early twenties: Less Snapchat, loads of TikTok, quite a bit of Instagram.
* Late twenties: A little bit less TikTok and *loads* of Instagram – mainly posts about your running journey and the cat you got with your first serious partner.
* Early thirties: Unbelievable amounts of Instagram. Devoted to your holidays and your nights out. Maybe a kid or a dog gets added along the way. TikTok too (but you're panicking about it because you don't fully get it).
* Late thirties into your forties: Instagram but for showing off your kid, dog or house reno. TikTok (you *never* post) and, secretly, Facebook to see how badly your school friends are ageing.
* Forties and fifties: Instagram and Facebook.

★ Over 50: Proudly only Facebook. And you're probably using one of those phone covers that opens out like a book and has a little fastener and holds all your store cards alongside a photo of your grandchildren. I am describing my mum here.

Horrible generalisations aside, I feel like we should have an ageing pep talk. My main message is 'your age is meaningless'; if nothing else, I hope by this point in the book I've made that clear. I'm celebrating my fortieth birthday this year and it's not sending me into a spiral of despair or making me veer into a crisis (yet). I feel happier, healthier and more connected to the world now than I did when I was 20. Big whoop, well done me. But it still feels important to say. You don't start decaying when you hit 25, despite what some would have you believe. The idea is to keep improving, keep learning and keep being interested in the world around you (developing a manageable skincare regime doesn't hurt either). I'm so done with being told what '40' means by other people that I'm in two minds about whether to even mark it. The way I've grown up seeing other people celebrate this milestone usually consists of either really owning it; having a huge party strewn with balloons that say YOU'RE 40! and buying a sports car (not no on that one). Or going the other way, ignoring it for as long as possible and trying to get away with being 39 for a few years. I think there's a third option. On the day itself, have a long bath while you drink wine and watch *Curb Your Enthusiasm*, then go out to dinner with your favourite people. This is currently where my head is, it sounds fitting.

Arbitrary age brackets play nicely into the very loud narrative on social media about what generation you're part of and (despite my silly social media age brackets earlier) I really hate being rounded up and shoved into a generational group. It's reductive, always leading to idiotic generation wars where people get so defensive and protective over a *made-up set of boundaries*. It's reached the point where I've started seeing millennials making being a millennial their *entire* personality, doubling down on tropes and fiercely defending the year they were born. This sort of boring shit just encourages people to carry on the age-old 'everything was better in my day' nostalgic nonsense.

Not every new thing is a threat or a replacement to the old thing or the old way. Nostalgia is brilliant sometimes, for sure. Songs, films and TV shows from our early and teenage years will always have special memories attached. But the new doesn't erase that. Kids aren't stupid for watching YouTubers or having a favourite content creator. Every generation has their things. Some of those will be shit and some fantastic – it's always been this way. Watching Mr Beast is just the current iteration of *CD:UK* or *Live & Kicking*, which was my favourite show when I was a lazy Saturday-morning slob child parked in front of the telly. Amelia Dimoldenberg's funny interviews are being enjoyed in the same way I might have watched Simon Amstell on *Popworld*, or Mr Shake Hands Man on *Banzai*.

I think it's important to find out what the new exciting things are before tutting disapprovingly. In doing so, you might just gain an understanding of why people like it. You might find you understand younger people more than you think. That might even make you like the world a bit more; you might lose that horrible feeling that it's leaving you behind.

The idea of evolving, of changing your tastes and your opinions is crucial to being an active member of society. Yes, it can be uncomfortable when you feel slightly out of touch with something but it's not a big task to give it a watch, listen to that new album everyone's going on about or just ask someone! Ask your kids, ask your nieces and nephews, ask the 20-year-old you work with. No one knows everything automatically; we all have to be taught at some point. I understand that naturally we all feel safer just sitting with the stuff we grew up with, and of course there are moments where I'll dive into Maxïmo Park's brilliant debut album from 2005 and be transported back to a hot day sitting on the grass at university, my fringe straightened, looking like a proper indie tragic, not worrying about anything – but that's not the *only* thing I listen to. I'm not committed to my 'own' generation's culture, refusing to move on.

This isn't to say that you have to like everything new. There's no need to force yourself to attend a Benson Boone show and start using the word 'sigma' if you don't want to. You can be who you are and like all the things you've always liked – but don't be scared of the younger people you will encounter in life. You might find they introduce you to something new to love. Younger people aren't scary, or even much of a mystery. The quickest way to feel completely removed from the world is to ignore all the changes happening around you. I know several people who still dress the same as they did when they were 18 and think that the best things have already been invented and there's no way a better film will ever be made than the one they watched in 2009.

The age vs. stuff you *should* like discussion is something that features heavily in my day-to-day life, with listeners often getting in touch with me to say, 'I shouldn't be listening, I'm out of your target age group but I still love Radio 1.' My reaction is always the same: 'Good! Don't worry about it. You're not alone. You're doing life properly! You're listening to a thing *you like.*' It was decided that age was the thing that should draw the lines between the radio stations when they drew up the BBC Charter back in the fucking Middle Ages. Radio 1's remit is supposed to be for 15–29-year-olds. Fair enough. I get what that means. It's supposed to be hyper-focused on things that the majority of people in that age bracket are talking about, but what if you never want to stop being interested in that stuff? You mustn't feel bad for liking things that someone tells you you're too old for. Those distinctions are entirely made up by people who are scared of the new and want to hold you back with them for safety in numbers. Also, the stuff a 15-year-old likes tends to be very different to the stuff a 29-year-old likes, and also no two 15-year-olds or 29-year-olds are the same.

My job has positively influenced the way I approach new ideas and culture. I get so much out of spending time with newer, younger producers and presenters, whether that's them sharing specific things they're into or their take on current world events, or simply being energised by their ambition and excitement for the place where we work. I love that I'm constantly exposed to brand-new music, brand-new ideas and brand-new ways of living your life. Like many millennials, I grew up in an age when being who you truly are wasn't celebrated in the way that it is now. I marvel at the bravery of teenagers proudly coming out as gay or trans or identifying as something other than a man or a woman. I feel in awe of young people who just know that they're bisexual and refuse to be shoved in one box or another. One week they've had a mad date night with Danny, the next they're on a wholesome weekend away with Leila. This would have blown my mind in 2000s Bishop's Stortford, and it's sad to realise how much mockery it would have provoked back then. I mourn my own teenage years a bit when I see younger people demanding to live as they choose, because they were pretty conservative and one-dimensional. To see the change in 20 years feels like huge progress. I realise there's a horrible irony at the recent Supreme Court ruling that trans women aren't legally women, but what the fuck does that even mean? You're whoever the hell you know yourself to be. It's a backwards step, and another reminder that we all have to try to understand the world as it changes.

Refusing to open your mind to new experiences ages you faster than anything else. But it also means you'll be constantly looking over your shoulder, reminiscing about 'the glory years' and feeling sort of permanently sad that those days are gone forever. Those glory days have been rose-tinted; even your memory of them has been smoothed and filtered and warped. You're remembering a time that didn't really exist. Life didn't peak with your last youthful day, whenever that supposedly was. It's good to embrace the way people, society and trends evolve. Except the Apple dance. I draw the line at the Apple dance. Despite everyone at work begging me to do it. No one needs to see that. I'll leave that to Charli.

Woke Nonsense!

I fall into the nostalgia trap all the time. I spent an hour watching old clips of early 2000s wrestling yesterday. I should have been writing this book but instead I watched The Rock vs. Stone Cold Steve Austin at WrestleMania 17. It was an amazing fight, by the way. Vince McMahon screwed The Rock over. Incredible drama. I sent one of the clips to my best mate Will who used to organise sleepovers at his house when there was a pay-per-view LIVE from America which inevitably finished at 3am. 'The old days WERE better, look!' I said to him in the accompanying message. But I didn't really mean that. What I really meant was, 'I love the memories of sitting around eating crisps and watching wrestling with you when we were teenagers and how carefree we were. I love how much we got into it. How nerdy we were about the staging, the pyro, the entrance music, the special effects, how the storylines were written and we were completely obsessed with the video montages they made to show in the pre-fight build up. They used to set these to the grungy American band of the moment and the best one ever was the promo for Rock vs. Austin at that WrestleMania. It was set to Limp Bizkit's 'My Way' and still makes my spine tingle when I watch it – which is at least once every few months.

Most of the things from past eras really aren't better, though. WWE (World Wrestling Entertainment, formerly WWF before the pandas kicked off about sharing a name) is a pretty handy barometer of where society is, and recently, there's been a very public reckoning for the company and more specifically, Vince McMahon, the co-founder and the man essentially responsible for it becoming a global phenomenon. He's been accused of enabling the sexual abuse of children (which he denies), and was at the helm when wrestlers were exploited, badly cared for, encouraged to work through injury and subjected to such busy schedules that some of them would wrestle 300 days a year while travelling around America. Painkiller and steroid addiction made many of them incredibly unwell and tragically contributed to ending careers and even some of their lives far too soon. As well as this, the attitude to women within the company has completely changed in the space of 20 years. I grew up as an impressionable teenager watching as women in the wrestling world were genuinely called the 'WWE Divas' and would be made to parade around in bikinis, called 'sluts' regularly, objectified by the wrestlers, the bosses, the commentators and therefore the crowd. At one point they were asked to play the role of sex workers that would accompany a wrestler called the Godfather. His 'shtick' was that he literally played the role of a 'pimp' and they were referred to on family television as his 'hoes'. I had to double-check these things happened and to my horror, they did. Today in WWE, there is an incredibly strong women's roster, genuine superstars who are celebrated and respected in-ring performers and not just used for punchlines and decoration. Whether forcibly or not, it had to move with the times.

This is how it should be. I hope everyone involved feels suitably uncomfortable about what they portrayed on screen because it definitely had an impact on millions of young people. I'm embarrassed that I saw it as entertainment now. It reduced women purely to their looks and firmly reinforced the lie that they were second-class citizens to the men that were in control. And although I had enough brilliant women in my life growing up to make sure that my only frame of reference for male/female relationships wasn't just weird ageing men on steroids ogling at tits and laughing, I was still affected by it, whether knowingly or not.

Attitudes towards people that are different have changed seismically over the last few years. Exacerbated by the constant flow of information online, we have a greater insight into people less fortunate than us, more fortunate than us and everyone in between. Nostalgia can be a false friend when you feel overwhelmed by 'keeping up with the times'. You see it every now and again when a newspaper or a website runs photos from the Victorian era, or the Second World War, and the comments inevitably say things like 'the good old days'. Ah yes, the good old days of rampant infant death, only upper-class white men having the right to vote and a WORLD WAR. What these comments really mean is that they feel some kind of nostalgia for a time long gone, just like I did when I sent Will old wrestling clips. It's an illusion, but it's a powerful one.

The world sometimes moves at what can feel like an alarmingly fast pace and some things that might've been said ten years ago are not acceptable now. Lessons we all have to learn about bias and bigotry can be hard and uncomfortable, but that doesn't mean we should turn away from them. Sometimes it doesn't feel like it, but largely things are moving in the right direction. I look back at some of the things I said at school and even on my early radio shows and wince. This isn't a nice feeling, but it is crucial to make sure you're growing as a person. Accepting that things change as the world moves on is alarming and sometimes destabilising but it is on all of us (if you're open-minded and decent) to be open to changing your opinions and viewpoints and admitting that you're wrong sometimes. The whole point of being alive is to try to get a little bit better at it every day.

You won't be right all the time. No one will. I don't have it sorted, by the way. I make mistakes, I still choose badly, I'm capable of being rude and unthinking sometimes. It would be weird if I wasn't. What *has* changed is being much more aware of those moments and learning the tools to navigate my way out of them fairly quickly. I have a much better sense of who I am and have managed to find a sort of default setting. And I've worked really hard with family, friends and co-workers to recognise where my blind spots are and how to undo them. If you're going to be a grown-up, you need to be open to the idea that you'll make mistakes. You must have the capacity to change, even if it feels hard at the time.

And sometimes it can be *really* hard. The advent of social media means you can be pulled up on your mistakes quickly and aggressively. There's a long-running joke that Twitter is a place where every day, the pack chooses one person to throw bottles at and you have to work hard not to be the person everyone's aiming at. Recently, I became the main character on Twitter for the day for a mistake I wish hadn't happened but I felt it was important to apologise and take responsibility for the offence it caused. There was a very unfortunate mistake on the announcement video for my children's book *The Twits Next Door*. I'm still deeply sad about this whole episode. Unfortunate is the best word for it and while I'm not writing this to excuse what happened, I'm putting it down here to tell you that as well as making sure you remember your childlike joy, sometimes you have to front up and be the most grown up you've ever been. Life can't always be fun. Particularly if you've upset lots of people: sometimes you just have to hold your hands up. My main mission with everything I make is to ensure people have a nice time and feel included. The opposite had happened here, we'd managed to make people who already felt excluded and marginalised feel even more so. My co-author Chris and I were gutted. We still are. I've since taken a lot of time to read up on this issue because despite making a mistake with the launch, it's clear my knowledge was lacking.

One of the strange bits of fallout from that rubbish day was hearing from a couple of well-known celebrities who would certainly class themselves as being 'cancelled by the woke mob'. Little did they know that I really like the woke mob. I don't know if I'm in it, but I'm certainly not angry with the idea of it. As I received these messages, it made me think about how easy it would have been to double down on the mistake we'd made and get angry about it. I forwarded one of them on to a mate of mine, saying, 'ONE OF US! ONE OF US! ONE OF US!' I wasn't going to fall for it. I joked with Bella a few days later about how in some ways people online go mad when they've fucked up. There's loads of examples of this, each of them a cautionary tale. People with amazing careers who in some cases have changed popular culture and garnered hundreds of millions of fans around the world with the things they've created get called out once for something they've done or said and instead of apologising or asking themselves some probing questions, they decide it's the hill they're willing to die on.

We all have to accept that we're going to mess up, upset people and get things wrong occasionally. And when we do, there are a couple of ways to approach it. We can really interrogate ourselves, ask whether we might have ballsed up, and consider how we might make things better. Or we can decide to stick to our guns and try to explain where we were coming from. As adults, we all have that choice. But we can't do what toddlers do and throw ourselves on the floor screaming, argue until we're blue in the face and refuse to take any blame. Well you can, but you'll be doing yourself a disservice. As kids, we're constantly told to grow and learn as much as possible. What kind of person wants to hit adulthood and stop doing those things?

I don't know what possesses people to choose option two. Just say sorry, for fuck's sake. I know Elton says it seems to be the hardest word but take some accountability and realise when you're making people feel sad, miserable and left out. The thing I find most baffling is why, when people make a mistake, they decide to recommit to punching down. Whether that's targeting trans people or an ethnic minority, or just decrying the 'wokerati', why choose that out of all the actual issues in the world you could make a positive difference with? I don't get it. Get over yourself and find something else to do. Maybe that's it! Get a new Dobby! Sorry, I mean hobby.

Long
Boi

OK. Rant over. Shall we return to some nonsense? I didn't think my life would ever lead to a moment where I'd be conducting a live memorial service for a duck on *The Radio 1 Breakfast Show*, but I'm glad it happened. Perhaps you haven't heard about Long Boi before. If so, your life is about to get 25 per cent better. Long Boi was Britain's tallest duck. An Indian Runner duck, he stood at an impressive 72cm tall. A beautiful boy. A lovely boy. A long boi.

I've long been obsessed with funny animal stories. I've created several features on the radio and the current iteration on the *Breakfast Show* at the time of writing is 'Animal News', which is just an excuse to talk about that badger who broke into a Superdrug a few years ago or the amazing dog that speaks Italian. By far the most extraordinary animal story I've ever come across is that of Long Boi. He lived – and loved – in the ponds at the University of York. He was and probably always will be the most famous thing about the university. The politician Harriet Harman, the author Anthony Horowitz and the comedian Harry Enfield all studied there but they are nobodies in comparison to our recently departed duck. We have talked about this guy a lot on the *Breakfast Show*. Why? Well, ducks are inherently funny. But it was more than that. He brought people together because people are united by wanting to have a nice time. And by knowing about the tallest duck in Britain, they felt like part of a club. Long Boi became the unofficial mascot for the university. He achieved worldwide fame, became the subject of countless memes, merchandise lines were created and sold on campus, he was included in welcome speeches to new students and graduation speeches for the old ones, and he gave me a good three years of content. For that alone, I'll be forever grateful.

I'd always wanted to meet him and had vowed to do my show from the side of the lake one day in an attempt to have him as a co-host. Life, as it tends to do, got in the way and tragically he went missing, presumed dead, before I got my shit together and made it to Yorkshire to see him. It will always be the biggest regret of my life. After several weeks of radio shows where we got people to go and look for him, take photos of potential ducks that could be him, we accepted this guy was a goner.

In an attempt to process the nation's collective grief, we started a search for Britain's next-tallest duck. It was a flop. We found a couple that barely scraped 60cm and an absolutely disgusting thing called Quaxel that Matlock Farm Park put forward for consideration. Honestly, to this day, I hate that fucking thing. Ugly as sin. A face that could haunt a house. He possessed nothing like the star quality our Long Boi did. It's always the way though, isn't it? The good die young. How is it fair that Long Boi's gone and kids have to put up with Quaxel strutting around Matlock? There's no justice in the world. Go on, google him. You'll see how weird he is. Yes, we should *care* for all animals but we don't have to *like* them all. At this point, the lawyers have requested that for balance

I thank Matlock Farm Park for their willingness to be on the radio and to remind readers that the award-winning Matlock Farm Park is the ideal place to visit to enjoy the fresh air of the countryside, combined with fun indoor and outdoor interactive experiences with a wide range of friendly animals. There is also a popular licensed café, a coffee shop and other takeaway catering outlets for refreshments during the day. And for a limited time only, you can take advantage of their 'Weekday Saver Deal' where up to two toddlers under the age of five GO FREE!

On the subject of animals I don't like, there's one in Dundee that I also hate. When we did Radio 1's Big Weekend there a few years ago, I'd heard that there was an anxious anteater in a nearby zoo that needed to be taken into consideration when we put on a horribly loud festival basically in its garden. I thought it would be really great to go and see it and meet the keepers, to thank them for being so welcoming of us all. Also, I'd never hung out with an anteater before so I was excited. The excitement was immediately dampened when I entered its weird little shed. A bucket of yoghurt had to be thrown in so that Nala, aged 17, would be distracted when we got near her. Apparently she can get quite violent. 'Oh,' I said out loud. I assumed an anxious diabetic (oh yeah, that too) anteater would be a little more welcoming of kindly visitors. This wasn't the case. I was told I could give her a little stroke. I wasn't keen but I didn't want to let the lovely keepers down so I obliged. It was like touching an old broom. Nala flinched slightly as she was slobbering away at the yoghurt with her giant hooter. The keeper was on edge. Nala was nervous. I was nervous. No one was having a nice time so I retreated. I noticed on the way out that she had her own broadband box set up in the shed which was linked to one of those diabetes things humans have on their arms. This mad creature with a hoover stuck on its face has got better Wi-Fi and healthcare than my nan. I started to resent the anteater so I thought it best to leave. I wish it no ill whatsoever but manners cost nothing and it would do well to remember that the next time an international radio star comes to visit.

Back to my glorious duck friend then. Long Boi's memorial came about after several months of discussion on the radio about how we could best honour his memory. The university decided that a statue should be erected near the pond he lived in. This was my opportunity to make amends. And to add that little showbiz sparkle to his life. One morning I declared that when the statue was ready to be unveiled, I'd do the *Breakfast Show* live from campus and conduct a fully live state funeral. It's the least I could do for this magnetic little guy.

I use the word magnetic without any irony. There is a reason 700 students wanted to get up early on a rainy Thursday morning in September to watch the tall idiot from the radio in full mourning-widow attire, complete with veil and sexy lace gloves, conduct a funeral for a dead bird. Silliness is the obvious reason. It's silly. And silly is my favourite thing. It's a great in-joke for those that know. The Long Boi club is a really good club to be part of. And of all the things I've ever done on the radio in my life, I put this at the very top. I've talked a lot about making sure we all put aside some time to remember the things that make us who we are. The fundamental things that we loved as children are probably the things we would love as adults. I'd have loved to have listened to someone conducting a funeral for a duck on the radio when I was a teenager. That whole event felt like the sort of thing I'd have done on student radio when I was 19. I wouldn't have been able to do it very well, mind you. I'm so fortunate to have the backing of a very famous and powerful radio station and the support of the best radio brains in the business. But creatively it felt closest to the 'oh fuck it, let's give it a go' spirit you tend to have when you're a fearless carefree teenager. And although we can't just dance through adult life doing that every day, it is possible to return to that blissful state more often than you probably realise. Ask yourself this, dear reader: what's *your* duck funeral?

I enjoyed every second of that memorial show. The build-up featured the university's vice-chancellor, Charlie Jeffery (incredible radio voice) talking about the impact of Long Boi on the culture of the campus, a chat with the sculptor – a very talented man called Neil Mason, and an appearance from Zoe, the person in charge of Long Boi's Instagram account which now boasts close to 60k followers. Without her, I don't think we'd have even heard of this majestic creature. The service itself started at 9.30 that morning and I mournfully walked across from our outside broadcast truck to the stage in the building opposite called Central Hall. This is the place that hosts end-of-year exams and graduation ceremonies. But on that drizzly autumn morning, it became a place of worship. And quacking. I took to the stage and read out my eulogy. I don't know if a duck eulogy has ever been published by a major publishing house so if not, you're holding history. A Duck and a Penguin in harmony.

I began:

Donald. Daffy. Daisy, Scrooge Mc. Just a few examples of ducks in popular culture that have made a global impact. And yet there's one duck that has transcended them all. He did it without the backing of either the Disney Corporation or Warner Brothers. And he did it without even trying. Some ducks just have it. And my god did Long Boi have it. He had it all.

He was the people's duck. Loved by all and yet ... a humble boy, a kind boy, a Long Boi.

Many of us saw ourselves in Long Boi. He was the best of us. He made the long-necked feel seen. He made the lanky heard. Publicly, he led a life of super-stardom and adoration – but in the pond, he reminded us of the harsh realities of life. Remaining stoic in the face of mockery by the more conventionally attractive birds. This only made us love him more. And the bullies, less. They were just jealous. And there was a lot to be jealous of.

My greatest sadness in life is that I didn't get around to seeing him before he passed. I will regret this for the rest of my days. But let this be a reminder to you all. Make the call, plan the trip, check in with those you hold dear. Whether it's a duck or a grandparent with questionable views on immigration. Pick up the phone, or bird feeder, and spend some precious moments with them. Because you never know when their time in life's great pond will be up.

So, thank you Long Boi. Thank you for the memes, the memories and the several years of Breakfast Show *content. We owed you this day.*

All the best for the future

I then proceeded to read out the Lord's Prayer which I'd re-written with the duck in mind. I didn't tell anyone back at Radio 1 HQ that I'd done this because I knew someone would panic and veto it.

Our Long Boi, who art in Yorkshire,
Legendary be thy name.
Your bill be gone,
Your quacking done,
Heard in York but now in Heaven.
Give us this day your daily bits of bread,
And forgive us hoisins,
As we forgive those hoisinned against you.
Feed us not into temptation,
But deliver us from Ed Gamble,
For thine lake is the kingdom,
Your long neck the glory,
For ever and ever,
Our friend.

A couple of things to add here. The Ed Gamble reference is because there was a strong rumour that he ate Long Boi on an episode of *The Great British Menu*. He has never denied this and in fact fanned the flames of it by saying he'd like to eat Pudsey from Children in Need and then my dog. He's a fucking monster and isn't to be trusted. That said, I do really like his podcast *Off Menu*. The other thing to add is that obviously I got the idea of the Lord's Prayer re-write because I realised I could do a play on words with hoisins and our sins. Some lovely low-hanging fruit. Here's a lesson: sometimes it's OK to do that. Low-hanging fruit can be delicious.

After the formalities, the university's Sing Song Society shuffled onto stage next to the cloaked bronze statue and sang a version of Chappell Roan's 'H-O-T-T-O-G-O' that had been re-written by a listener called Megan to 'L-O-N-G-B-O-I'. I can't say this enough – the listeners are the reason I wake up and feel excited about going into work every day. Megan called up the show excitedly to tell me about this. And it's genius. The brilliant breakfast team, consisting of Amy, Thom, Susanna and Vinuri, then set about writing the rest of the verses and chorus, gave it to the choir and they practised it quickly. It was an extraordinary team effort. In less than 48 hours it had gone out live on Radio 1 to millions of people, then went viral on TikTok and was featured on the *BBC News at Six*. It was incredible. They then sang Wiz Khalifa's 'See You Again' and I pulled the sheet off the bronze duck and there he was. A loud gasp echoed around the auditorium. It was weirdly emotional. I announced we'd commence a minute of quacking. And for a glorious 60 seconds, a radio station that once had The Beatles playing live, was on air during the fall of the Berlin Wall and broadcast the Queen's funeral was now home to 700 adults quacking at a statue. It will forever be my proudest moment. We all decamped to the lake and when I got there, the path was lined with hundreds of students waiting for a ceremonial Viking burial. It was so busy. In my memory, it looked as full as The Mall at the Queen's Diamond Jubilee when everyone came out to watch Gary Barlow do that song with the choir and Andrew Lloyd Webber. As an aside, I just fact-checked that on YouTube and that segment was introduced by the convicted sex offender Rolf Harris. We had a very strict 'no sex offenders' policy at our event but we did put a call out and two Norse lads from the Jorvik Viking Centre turned up to help me push an inflatable duck raft out into the pond where Long Boi lived. I wanted to go the whole hog and set fire to it like they did in those days but sadly the BBC were worried we might burn down a swan by mistake.

Yes, the whole thing was stupid but for one morning, we were all playing. And it was so much fun. It was grown adults messing around making something silly for the sake of it. The atmosphere was friendly and people were brought together; I made hundreds of new friends and got to know the university staff really well. It was a celebration of teamwork, of nothing being bigger than the sum of its parts, and of animals. The joy of animals. When you have an opportunity to celebrate just one of those things, let alone all of them, you should take it. And we all took it that day. And threw everything at it. We were all part of a community. A daft one, but a community nonetheless. That duck brought us all together, made us forget about our troubles for a morning and we were reminded of the lighter side of things. The light exists even in the sadness. You might have to search really hard for it, but it's always there. And it usually involves other people. And that's what we all want, isn't it? To feel part of something. Recently, I was part of the now legendary gig at the O2 when Pitbull entertained 20,000 fans with a night of pure bangers. Most of the crowd, as I'm sure you heard, were dressed up as him. It was a sea of bald heads bobbing up and down. It was pure joy. We're all desperate to share experiences together, to be part of something, and for the night, we were in the Pitbull gang. Just like in York we were in the Long Boi gang. A shorthand for nonsense. Thinking about it, Pitbull would have loved Long Boi. Game recognising game. Or in this case, game recognising dog. So whether it's dressing up as Mr 305 and swinging your partner round and round to 'Timber', or on the banks of a river clapping a dead duck – life's better when you share it. And it's definitely better if you're laughing. Pitbull's laughing. Laughing all the way to the bloody bank after taking my suggestion to sell his own branded bald caps and glasses at his shows seriously. No cut for me. That's showbiz!

The day after the memorial service, my agent received an email from Big Boss Aled at Radio 1 offering me another year on the *Breakfast Show*. I laughed out loud at the timing. Must have been the hoisins bit.

Worrying
About
Worrying

L ife would be great if it was all Long Boi and fun stuff, wouldn't it? Imagine how great it would be if you could stop worrying. Alas, it's impossible, but you can take great comfort in the fact that every single person worries about things. Big things, little things, stupid things, embarrassing things, boring things, actual things, completely made-up things. All humans worry. Here are some of the worries I've had in the last 39 years of my life. Some of them have an age associated with them. Those left ageless indicate I *still* worry about them. These won't leave me until I die.

Am I too tall?

Am I ugly?

Will anyone ever fancy me? 12–18

What if I get sacked from Radio 1? 21–24

How the fuck do you know if you should marry the person you're having sex with? 17–33

What if my parents suddenly die in the night (and I wake up a sad orphan)?

Am I weird for not wanting a girlfriend? 9–17

Who am I?

Will people laugh at me if I tell them I volunteer at hospital radio? 15

Is it weird that I don't want kids?

Am I boring?

Is this book boring?

Why don't I like football more than I do?

What if I never like beer? 7–17

Am I depressed or just a bit sad? 27–33, 36 (basically, through-out the pandemic)

Why do people get so serious during sex?

Am I going to die alone?

When will I get cancer?

Will it be bad cancer?

Am I thick?

What *are* my hobbies?

Am I losing hair at the temples? 38

What if I can't exercise anymore?

What clothes are good?

What if I lose my voice or my hearing?

What if this hand dryer I'm using blows up? (I really hate hand dryers. Why are they so loud? All that screaming. Hideous inventions. And yeah, the intrusive thought is that they will explode in my face and result in life-altering injuries. I think that is totally rational.)

As you can see. It's a real mix of things. BIG worries mixed in with little ones. Most brains have the capacity to do this. The big worries coexist with the small ones, all of them taking up space in the same way, turning it into a vast anxious cavity. I find that extraordinary. Your mum might be seriously ill in hospital but your brain still allows you to think about how much of a rip-off the privately owned car park's going to be. This is a magnificent feat, and totally normal. I mean, I hope to God it's normal. There are people who have studied brains for years who still don't fully understand them, so go easy on yourself if yours confuses you from time to time. It's extraordinary that we live with a thing in our heads that we don't truly understand – but maybe that's the brain's ultimate trick – it can't understand itself. It's a bit like how you can't see yourself blinking.

Much like having your own podcast, iced lattes and hearing world leaders say racist things every day, discussing mental health has become much more mainstream in the last few years. This is largely a good thing because people have a brain and therefore being aware of how to treat it well is vital to your survival. 'Mental illness' when I was growing up was something that happened to other people and you wouldn't think twice about saying someone had been 'carted off to the loony bin' or something equally flip-pant. 'Breakdowns' were seen as a weakness or even something to be laughed at or mocked. Depression was considered the result of bad life choices, and anxiety was something you thought you had if you were a bit worried about your GCSE mocks. It's embar-rassing that it's taken so long to change. Imagine how many lives would have been improved and saved if everyone had wised up and realised that brain health is just as important as everything else.

'Mummy, are we panicking yet?' is a phrase that has haunted me my entire life and yet I only ever said it once. I remember the moment vividly – Mum and I were rushing along the platform at Waterloo Station for a train to Weymouth to see Nan and Gran-dad. I must have been about six years old and we were about to miss our train. As the fast walking turned to jogging which then became running and finally sprinting, I realised something was up.

It's the first memory I have of my mum losing her composure. It was the first chink I detected in her usually calm and unflappable demeanour as we hurtled across the concourse and she replied, 'Yes! We're bloody panicking. Now come on!' Big moment. Huge moment. The safety net was giving way. There was a split in the webbing! What do you do when the safety net frays?! I remember being so unbelievably anxious and worried at that moment, to this day I still think about it every time I'm catching what I'd call a 'big train' out of London. But on that day, even though the safety net showed signs of ripping, it didn't and we made the train. Only just, though. But even if we hadn't made it, I wouldn't have had to solve the problem, my mum would have done it somehow. That's one of the joys of a safe and secure upbringing and if you're lucky, you had one. I did. I was lucky. It's not about pretending life doesn't get rough sometimes, it's more about someone being there to catch you when you fall. Sometimes literally.

And then you grow up. As an adult, you are your own safety net and – even more frighteningly – you're also probably part of someone else's. The worries I experienced in early life were just illusions of worry. If you're fortunate, someone will be worrying on your behalf and will help solve the problem before it gets too severe. It's a bit like when you're learning to drive and the instructor has a set of pedals on their side to stop you running over a sluggish pensioner on a zebra crossing. We're not necessarily equipped to deal with worry and sadness when they affect us. We're always being told to 'talk about it', but who do we talk to? And how do we explain what's going on inside our brains, when we barely understand ourselves? We're constantly pushed the idea of 'finding happiness' and I have to say, in my old age, I've grown suspicious of 'happiness' as a concept. It's also turned into a huge industry, riddled with grifters and people who can promise you a better life, a one-way ticket to the promised land! But really it's a front to get you to buy their dodgy supplements or self-help plan (just £15.99 a month!) or worse, their week-long wellness retreat. But what does 'a better life' mean? Let's be blunt about it: the basics of a 'good adult life' should be 1) enough money to be comfortable, 2) a roof over your head and 3) staying in good health. If you've got those things, you're one of the lucky ones. Beyond that, the 'happiness goal' is nonsense.

No one has ever or will ever be happy the entire time. It isn't a destination that you can get to and trying to reach it is a trap many of us fall into. 'If I meet the right person, get the right job and buy the right car I'll *finally* be happy!' I'm not saying happiness doesn't exist, I'm just here to remind you that it comes and goes and that's completely normal. What I've come to realise is that it's *contentment* we should be looking for. Life becomes a lot less overwhelming when you stop trying to look at it as a continuous game that if you play well you'll get to the promised land of 'Happy'. It's a lot simpler than we realise. It might not be as satisfying to learn that you can't achieve 'Ultimate Happiness Level 10' but what I find more exciting and rewarding is that there are endless moments of joy and contentment to be found along the way. I'm not even talking about big new jobs or swanky holidays; I'm interested in the little bits of joy that help the day skip past. You have to have your eyes open to find it all, by the way. Sometimes you have to be really willing to see it. For example,

I find it a lovely and peaceful moment when I'm accompanying my dog outside at 5am so that he can go for a piss before I leave for the *Breakfast Show*. There's no one around. Just me and this ridiculous creature that lives in our house who just wants to have a nice time. Barney's a great advocate for contentment. He doesn't give the path of his life a second thought. He's existing fully in each minute of the day, looking for the next bit of fun or food. We can learn a thing or two from that. Humans have much more complicated brains and we don't (usually) shit in the street so you have to try much harder than he does to find the contentment. Another nice part of my routine after I've watched my dog piss is waving at Josephine who opens up the little Tesco near me as I cycle to work every morning. She has a beaming smile and I ding my bell (not a euphemism) and give her a shout as I trundle past with my eyes barely open. I know these things sound a bit daft but they help distract me from the simple fact that I do not want to be up at that time. I might be doing my dream job but I still think it's awful to get up at 5am, so you have to make it nice for yourself in whatever way you can.

If Bella or I have had a shit day or some bad news or we're stressed and tired, we'll ask each other if there's a way to make the day beautiful. This is the cheesiest we get but it works. It's usually solved by a walk with Barney as the sun sets, a trip to the shop to get some chocolate or just loads of wine. There seems to be a notion that your life will only properly start when you've reached this nebulous 'Happy Place'. Don't be fooled by that; your life is *live* right now, so don't wait for the 'next level' because you'll forget to enjoy the moment you're living in. Refocus on those and

All the best for the future

I don't think you can go too far wrong but also, be realistic and go easy on yourself. Life is really hard most of the time, even if you've got your shit together, and being responsible for your own mental wellbeing can sometimes seem like a Herculean task. I exercise, I try to get enough sleep, eat the right amount of vegetables, pop vitamins until I rattle, I see my friends as often as possible and wrestle with Barney every other day. But sometimes none of it helps, none of it takes away the worries. None of it makes me truly happy because I don't think that exists. And I realise now I'm OK with that. Blimey, that last stretch could have been written by Pitbull. ¡DALE!

Look Out!

L ooking outwards is something I try really hard to do. To try to get out of my own brain. We can all become really easily self-obsessed – please welcome: Main Character Syndrome! It happens to us all. I'm pretty good at dishing out this advice to Bella, who is prone to bouts of anxiety, intrusive thoughts and OCD. Bella has written beautifully and honestly about her struggles with mental illness and her candidness around medication, which I know for a fact has helped many people over the years. The stigma around drugs to treat mental health issues, although waning, is still a huge barrier for people to get over. I try my best to help Bella by always trying to nudge her to 'look outwards' when she's in a particularly tough spot. This, of course, has to be done gently and sympathetically, but what I mean by this is reaching out for those things that bring you comfort or happiness or even safety. Like many people, she works alone. She is therefore at an immediate disadvantage because she doesn't have any colleagues in the vicinity. Apart from our dog, but he just sits there barking and farting. Yes, I hear you, that's preferable to some of the knobs you work with. But still, working with like-minded funny people is the thing that keeps me most sane. So I always try to remind Bella to stop work-ing every now and again and visit a friend or her mum just to break any unhelpful thoughts her brain is trying to obsess over.

I've talked a lot in this book about how technology and in particular social media simultaneously connects us to everything and everyone and yet can leave us feeling frighteningly alone. Therefore it's a really great idea to be on the front foot and seek out connection. This could be a friend or family member you haven't caught up with in a while, or on a more civic level, helping with something in your local area. I listened to a brilliant episode of *The Ezra Klein Podcast* recently where he talked about the perils of hearing the news from all corners of the world. It's of course important to keep up to date with as much as you can but he made the point that we're in danger of ignoring our immediate environment. Yes, you're up to date with everything Trump's said today (oh God!) but did you realise that the local library needs volunteers otherwise it's going to have to reduce its opening hours? Oh great, Putin's gone mad again, but also the old guy next door (not the anti-abortion guy, a lovely man called Tom on the other side) would have really liked a hand repotting some bulbs on his front path. There will be some brilliant local things you could get involved with instead of being obsessed with what someone the other side of the ocean is dancing to on TikTok. This bit of the book is a reminder to me as much as it is you as I really would like to go and volunteer at the primary school near me to see if they need any help reading to the kids. There's also a little farm nearby that I'm trying to get Bella to go and help out at. Refocusing on the world immediately around you is hard when we're constantly bombarded with things we're told to care about but might really add a lovely new dimension to your week.

Aside from these slightly less obvious ideas, exercise is nearly always a good idea to clear a fogged-up mind. I've been lucky that

I've always enjoyed sport and generally being active and I've been running since I was a teenager. I started jogging around regularly when I was about 15 and quickly got hooked on the idea of listening to my favourite music out of the house, away from my parents and homework as I darted off with my MP3 player blasting Linkin Park, Limp Bizkit or Avril Lavigne on the mean streets of Bishop's Stortford.

I found running to be a real escape for my brain, which has always had a tendency to overthink and rattle through thoughts at a terrifying rate. I've spent many years getting those traits to a place where they can serve me well, but they still paralyse me at times. I spoke to my parents about this recently and they confirmed that I was quite timid as a child. Moving around and having to start several new schools in a matter of just a few years didn't help things. New schools and new sets of friends take their toll on all kids to some degree but they were really worried for the first couple of terms at secondary school because I knew nobody there when I started and I would often not want to go. The hour-long bus ride full of kids from several different schools was particularly intimidating for me as I was in a new town, my mum and dad were both teaching at schools in different counties and there were no friends waiting for me at the other end. At least not at the beginning. Part of the upheaval of moving regularly meant that I had to get really good at being on my own and happy in my own company. I don't remember being particularly sad but I do have a recollection of wanting to feel a bit more like I belonged somewhere. Being good at cricket was a breakthrough for me because it became my 'thing', something I was known for, and gave me something to talk about with other kids who were cricket obsessed.

I've never been particularly confident with my looks or my body, particularly when I was younger. I really hated my body. I thought I was too lanky and too limby but at the same time quite doughy and cumbersome. I also didn't like my nose as it was too big and pointy for the rest of my face, and I thought my teeth were goofy. I would look at some of the other, sportier boys in my year with envy that they'd started filling out muscle-wise and were slowly becoming young men, whereas I still felt like a boy. Running was a real breakthrough for me and made me feel happy and peaceful – it still does. I love the feeling of my body being able to do that and it terrifies me that it might seize up one day and I won't be able to do all the things I love. In the last year or so, I've started to take my health and fitness a lot more seriously: partly due to being more aware of my own mortality and approaching middle age but also because during the pandemic, I slipped into what I would amateurishly describe not as depression but a depressed state where I stopped caring about my body and my mind and just went into a numb survival mode. I started to become sluggish, sleepy and unthinking about what I was feeding myself. I was easily distracted, irritable and unfocused on what I was even trying to achieve in my home life, let alone work. That's nothing special, by the way; millions of people around the world did this and we probably haven't fully come to terms with it yet.

I now recognise how damaging it is to talk derogatively about my body and have stopped thinking of it as something I want other people to be impressed by. *I* want to be impressed with what it can do, not what it looks like. Whereas once I might have longed for a six-pack, I have found a new way of being proud of my strength and agility instead. Now, I am extremely proud of how flexible I am thanks to yoga, I love that I can swim, run and cycle whenever I want. I can do long walks, climb hills and most importantly, pick up my large, very arthritic dog and carry him up and down stairs if he needs to. He's 35kg, by the way. Basically a small horse. I want to future-proof my body as well as I can, and exercise helps with that. Keeping everything well oiled and strong gets harder as you go on but can minimise the chances of ending up wandering around like the Tin Man, or getting out of breath at the most gentle of inclines.

The world has changed remarkably since our parents were our age. There's a load of very funny videos on TikTok of twenty- and thirty-somethings comparing their lives to the lives of their parents at the same age. Invariably, it's always a photo of their parents nicely settled down with a house and two kids compared to a photo of the chaotic millennial putting on a birthday party for their cats in their rented apartment. We tend to stay 'younger' for longer and although I'm well aware that anyone younger than a boomer finds it much harder to buy a house than them, this has forced people to investigate different ways to navigate life and disregard the yardsticks that previous generations have lived by.

When I was younger, I didn't give being 40 much thought but I didn't think it would be like this. It's really great, to be honest. I'm much happier now than I was at 20 or even 30, mainly because I've remembered all the things that I love and that bring me joy – but I've also gained confidence to still lean into them. Many of us are ageing in a different way, and this is progress! I love gardening but I also love going out and getting battered at gigs – and not just of the bands I liked when I was 18. I really love going to National Trust properties but also enjoy a truly debauched weekend at Glastonbury. I like old cars but still love watching *The Simpsons* while eating crisps. I love pushing myself to try on clothes that historically I'd have been too scared to; I like being surprised by a new album from an artist I've never heard of; I love learning about why people follow certain trends, finding out why Chappell Roan or Doechii are so adored; and on a deeper level, I love the relationship I have with my parents. It's far less formal than the relationship my parents had with theirs. My grandparents were *old people* my entire life; compared to what my parents look like now, you'd say my nan and grandad were 400 when in reality they were only in their early seventies. I'm genuinely mates with my mum and dad and that relationship brings me so much joy and comfort. I spend hours walking and chatting with my mum and days on end watching sport with my dad, and I imagine even they're surprised that they didn't just raise a son, but created a friend.

One of the joys of being an adult can be that you become friends with your parents. I'm sure a lot of you reading this are in that boat, and yes, it's a lucky boat but it also comes with its perils. This particular friendship has a unique intensity attached to it because if it all goes to the universe's plan, they will die within your lifetime. You'll likely outlive them by many years. The roles tend to reverse and you might well end up looking after them at the end of their lives, like they did for you at the start of yours. You're now giving the people that taught you about the world advice on how to live well, eat well, keep moving and stay connected to the world. They're entering a second childhood at the very moment you've begun to make sense of your adulthood.

I've mentioned that my dad's had health scares since I was a teenager but I always thought he'd bounce back as he was much younger. And thankfully, he did! They're both north of 70 now so obviously the potential for illness is greater, as is the likelihood that they'll find it more difficult to overcome it. That sentence is quite bleak but it's true, isn't it? A real worry for people that get on with their parents is them leaving you alone in the world. My mum only recently lost her mum. Nan was 100! Insanely old, and yet it still has had a profound impact on Mum. It's going to be sad whenever it happens, but the way I rationalise with myself is to think that any time you have with your parents after the age of 30 is a massive bonus. They did all they could for me and gave me the best start in life – no one can take that away from me. We're way into bonus territory here and if they were to disappear tomorrow, I'd of course be horribly sad but I would know that I made the very best of them and our relationship.

When we're young, we tend to be fearful, suspicious and even dismissive of ageing but when you get here, you realise it doesn't have to be a devastating slide into irrelevance. It's not even as if I'm fighting getting old; you just don't have to. Growing up and getting old is a trap and an easy one to fall into, so think about whether you want to.

Martha

The way I approach my day-to-day life changed dramatically in 2021 when a friend's daughter died very suddenly after an accident on holiday. Her death was entirely avoidable, a complete tragedy. Despite only meeting her a handful of times, I think about Martha often. She was 13 when she died in hospital of sepsis – which wasn't caught as early as it should've been. Merope, Martha's mum, had made me aware that she and her younger sister Lottie were avid Radio 1 listeners and had also enjoyed a few of my children's books. I later learnt that Martha herself was a sensational writer. It was a real joy to get to hang out with them both. Martha loved the word 'jolly'. Well, it's a funny-sounding word so who can blame her? Maybe because it sounds like jelly. And jelly is also funny. But Martha was jolly personified. I realised immediately that we shared a belief that there's always fun to be found and it's pretty much always a good idea to be silly and/or jolly, and eat jelly. In fact, her outlook on life is essentially what I've been talking about throughout this book. She knew at 13 how to approach life properly. It took me a little longer. It's perhaps because Martha was also devastatingly smart. Quicker than most adults in her orbit and she adored reading. On a recent catch-up with Merope, she reminisced that Martha was one of the few children in the world who had to be told to take a break from books every now and then. She would have no doubt gone on to create wonderful things with her phenomenal brain. It's brilliant that Merope and Paul, Martha's dad, have created the Martha Mills Young Writers' Prize in her honour. It celebrates curious and imaginative young writers and is a fitting way to keep her memory and spirit alive.

Of course, I'd realised that life was fragile long before Martha died so tragically. I knew nothing lasts forever. I knew that people died, and I knew how sad that could be. But all the people I'd lost that were close to me were old. They'd done things. They'd at least finished school, got pissed, rented a flat, gone away without their parents, seen the world, fallen in love, had their hearts broken and likely broken someone else's. Martha didn't get to do any of that and her death was a startling reminder that life isn't just fragile – it's also really cruel. Inexplicably mean and unjust. How do you square that with all the jolliness around? How do you simply 'carry on' with the mundane tasks, the work emails, opening letters from EDF fucking Energy, putting the bins out on a Tuesday night. What's the point of it all if everything can be taken away from you at any moment?

I hate EDF Energy. If I have to re-book another Smart Meter appointment because they keep demanding I have one but then fail to show up, I'm going to scream. But the answer is, you have to keep going. You just have to. Because the alternative is dreadful. You can't give up. The world is exhausting but maybe there's an expectation issue here. Are we making a mistake thinking that everything's going to work out just the way we want if only we work hard enough at it? Because it's difficult to hear, but the default setting in life isn't 'good'. The default, if we're lucky, is 'meh'. And maybe that's helpful somehow. Because it's a sort of halfway house. Below 'meh' is 'shit' but *above* 'meh' is 'good'. If you're living expecting everything to be good, then you're going to be disappointed quite often. But of course, if you live your life expecting everything to be shit, it might well end up shit and you'll be depressed. Living in the middle is much healthier and a lot calmer.

Life is long if you're very lucky. It undulates and it'll be tough a lot of the time. But is there some comfort that everyone is also having to come to terms with this too? My grief at Martha's death wasn't even remotely comparable to that of her parents, but I felt it nonetheless. And my way of trying to understand why this had happened to her was to realise there's actually nothing *to* understand. Trying to be rational is a waste of time in this instance. There is nothing anyone could ever say that could possibly make her death make sense. Not for me, not for her parents, not for her sister or her friends. It is just completely awful. The only way through is to realise that there is no plan for us. There are no guarantees. There's only luck and the inescapable fact that time marches on.

Growing up is maybe the process of understanding this, and being robust enough to deal with it. The unknown. The inexplicable. I now realise that what happened to Martha could happen to any of us at any time. No matter how young, fit, happy, successful or talented we are. So please stop worrying and fucking get on with it. If you understand that, I think that makes you a grown-up. That's the best explanation of the term. That's what maturity is. Not some arbitrary signal which might come in the form of a mortgage or a nice car. That's not maturity. That's cosplaying as an adult you've seen depicted somewhere. Being a grown-up is finding genuine peace that awful things always happen and realising that unfortunately some of them will happen to you, whether you deserve them or not. Once you've come to terms with this, you can hopefully control the bits of your life you're lucky enough to be able to. Plan that amazing trip, ask that person on a date, make the most of that gym membership. Do some things that bring you joy. Or don't! Sitting around not travelling or not going to the gym might be just what you need! Use Martha as inspiration to work out who you are and what makes you tick. She knew exactly who she was at 13, so you have no excuse! Just remember that your time is limited, just like mine, so don't take it for granted. If I ever find myself forgetting this, Martha will appear in my thoughts and remind me what a privilege it is to be able to plan for the future; I hope she'll appear in yours too. Now go off and do something jolly.

Just
Boring
Enough

When you're faced with something like a loss you realise that life is short, fragile and precarious and some people decide to act on this and write a list of the maddest things they can think of and go off to complete their bucket/fuck it lists. I get that. I really do. I have a list of things I want to do when I take my foot off the work accelerator a bit. Travelling the world is my main one. But is there also something to be said for embracing life in all its ordinary and mundane glory? Sometimes it's really good to embrace that really boring side of yourself.

A few weeks ago when sorting out car insurance renewals, I proudly said to Bella that I was just boring enough. When I turn it on, I'm really good at all the dull shit you have to do as an adult. By her own admission, she is not. When we first started going out, I'd have to wade through countless red-topped reminder letters from various utility companies that she'd forgotten to pay. People are different and that's great, but sometimes I was so stressed on her behalf that I would call British Gas and explain the situation. As I've said, I didn't grow up destitute but there was never any money spare, it would always have to be carefully placed and accounted for. I've inherited this very unsexy but useful trait, and despite being in a position where I could now throw money at a problem if needed, I try to remain true to my money-anxious roots and teachings. It's not just money- or bills-based, by the way. It applies to parking permits, maintenance, bins and a whole host of boner-killing logistics, as you're about to find out.

Bella is sitting opposite me for this bit of the book and is going to shout out boring things I do and I'm going to defend them.

You ordered a job lot of fire blankets and extinguishers

This was a response to Bella's sister nearly burning her house down with a candle, and I thought, *Why wouldn't you have a blanket in the kitchen?* As previously mentioned, one of my childhood heroes was Fireman Sam, and I thought, *What would he do?* Everyone thought Sam was cool; nobody ever said he was boring, did they? This reminds me to buy an even bigger one for the house, so you've helped me out here.

Insisting we replace our lovely old front door with a safer and uglier one

This isn't boring at all; it's a standard requirement for all sane people. I actually think this shows that you would rather have had a door made essentially of cardboard if it looked pretty. We had to have a new window put in and the guy said, 'You might as well not have a front door, you could push that one in through with one finger.'

Ordering bulk packs of dishwasher cleaner which take up a whole cupboard – ditto toothpaste and toilet paper

Again, this is just right. One of the most annoying things in the world is running out of toothpaste and toilet paper so this seems like a helpful thing to do for us. The dishwasher cleaner is an entirely separate matter; you have to stay on top of the maintenance of these machines. Treat them well, and they'll treat you in kind. They're doing the hard yards for you, so giving them a clean is the least you can do.

Having a family phone plan, which means I have to call you and ask you for more data

I'm not a tight man, and Bella, you will attest to this (she is nodding). I like having a nice time. And I like helping other people have a nice time. However, I turn into Ebenezer Scrooge when it comes to paying monstrous utility companies. I will sit on the phone with Sky for an hour just to make sure they're not ripping us off. So yes, every month, since I expertly negotiated unlimited data, I have to gift my wife some of it. Which leaves me more money to spend on dishwasher cleaner and toothpaste. Work smarter, not harder.

OK fine, but you once offered to get your mother-in-law a tyre inflator for Christmas – surely that crosses over the line into full boring

This is because she brought up that it would be a good idea to have a car full of emergency rations and basic maintenance gear. I told her I had all that stuff in my boot and that I even had a tyre inflator which plugs into the cigarette lighter. She was surprisingly enthusiastic and given that it was in the weeks leading up to Christmas, I thought it was only polite to offer her one. Let's not mention that the first time I used mine, I drained the battery. Nobody's perfect.

You got a Curzon cinema membership and gleefully calculated how often we had to go for it to be worth it

What's boring about culture, Bella? Sorry for wanting to expand our minds. What can I say? I like being part of a club. And if that club gives me five free tickets a year, even better. That being said, using the expression 'it pays for itself' is indefensible so I'll give you this one. Very boring.

OK then, how do you explain your mad obsession with the DVD player you bought?

It's BluRay, first of all, and this is another way to fight against 'the man'. And in this instance the man is the collective power of the streaming companies which means following your favourite shows around these platforms. We don't own anything anymore – they do. So buying the DVD player and stocking up on my favourite films and shows is my way of wrestling back some kind of power. Who's got the rights to *Curb Your Enthusiasm*? Doesn't matter, because I own physical copies and I can watch them whenever I fucking want. (Bella has since pointed out that this makes me sound like David Brent, and incidentally I also have the complete series boxset of *The Office* INCLUDING the Christmas specials on BluRay, so up yours, Amazon Prime.)

I'm going to win with this one. You spent days researching a tumble dryer and then showed it to guests when they came round

Like many boring things in my life, this started as a joke and then I got such a genuinely excited reaction from the first person I showed that the mask became the face and the tours became unironic. But again, treat your white goods with respect. And people seemed up for it when I offered them a first look. I'm a showman, I can sell anything.

You got a Tesco Clubcard despite never going to Tesco and then gleefully waved it at me when I did

Again this harks back to 'don't let the man fuck you over'. How dare supermarkets display two prices? Do I care enough to try to bring them down? No. I stop at the Clubcard; I can see it could be the end of my marriage if I got too obsessed with this injustice. But is my personal data worth sacrificing for one pound off Marmite? Fuck yes it is.

You're a really good driver but you spend whole journeys talking about other people's bad driving

Driving standards have slipped massively over the past 15 years. I genuinely consider being a good driver my greatest skill. This is also reflected in my TikTok algorithm which consists mainly of driving instructors and dashcam footage. My toxic trait is thinking I'd be an amazing traffic cop. Because I'm safe, but fast. Incidentally this is also an example of good pillow talk.

Mum said that the sexiest thing a man can do is pay the TV Licence

Was this your mum flirting with me? This annoyed me because it does sound boring on the surface. I want to be a mysterious cad! But she reassured me that you can be both, and then she told me I'm handsome. And your mum's a good-looking woman, so I'm happy with that. It's also a sackable offence at the BBC not to have a TV licence. Besides, it pays my wages.

I just want to point out here that I pay the TV Licence

That is true but we only have one TV in the house so that is ... that is fine. And thank you for paying my wages.

I've Been Busy Thinking About Boys

I've written about many important things in this book but this might just be the most important of all so I want you to listen carefully. *You'll probably never be happy with your hair.* It took me 35 years to nail how to do my hair properly, and then suddenly it went to shit. I was finally happy with the length, the way it sat on my head, the products I was using and then everything changed. My scalp started itching, the product didn't work in the same way, it was all fluffy. I was in a crisis. It's a good metaphor for life. Actually it's not good at all, but it *is* a reminder that just when you think everything's sorted and hunky dory, the world can have other plans for you.

I was born with a full nest of thick black hair which my mum often still talks about. Mums love talking about your hair when you were a baby. I've been shown the photos and what I see is not a sweet toddler with an amazing mane of hair but more a marrow (they're green, by the way) in a cheap black wig. I have an irregular-shaped head. It is like an upturned watermelon, or weirdly, a marrow. The wrong cut for me can be a disaster. Whenever I'm asked if I'd ever go skinhead or buzzcut, I'm forced to reply, 'I don't have the head for it, dear!' while miming taking a puff of a cigarette like a fabulously camp actress from the 1930s. I really *don't* have the head for it, though. Northern Neil who cuts my hair says to me that I have a head like a 50-pence piece. All jaggedy and irregular. I've always been told it's a watermelon or a marrow and *now* you're telling me the surface is uneven? Which is it, Neil?! It's always lovely to pop in and see him for a self-esteem pick-me-up every few weeks. He's not wrong, though; a quick google of me over the years will show some absolute horrors where my hair just doesn't look right. You might not know what I'm talking about at all with this and you've probably never given my hair a first thought, let alone a second (and fair enough), but my obsession with it is a perfect example of the madness of human adults. You'll have a hang up about something and I bet none of your friends would go, 'Oh yeah, I've always thought that about you.' It's invariably something that exists solely in (or on) your own head.

Bella has banned me from talking about my hair with her, so I'm afraid you're going to have to be my audience for this madness. Embracing your hang-ups and being honest with your-self about them is incredibly healthy (that's what I'm telling myself at least). Even the most 'together' grown-ups will have many, *many* unhinged thoughts about themselves, and the sooner you realise that we're all a bubbling mess of insecurities and mad thoughts, the better.

There's a photograph of me, aged 17, taken at a sixth-form induction day that I think about far too often. It still makes me physically shudder every single time, even 20 years later. I went to an all-boys secondary school in Bishop's Stortford, imaginatively named 'The Bishop's Stortford High School' or TBSHS for short, but saying TBSHS is way more complicated and takes longer than using its full name. Despite Years 7–11 being single sex, the sixth form … deep breath … LET GIRLS IN! Holy fucking Christ, this was a seismic moment for the hundreds of nervous, anxious, horny boys. Full panic mode set in on our induction day. Those of us who didn't hang out with girls that much just didn't know what to do or how to play the next couple of years and the whole thing still gives me nightmares. The photo that still haunts me perfectly sums up that time. It's of me and my best mate, Will. We're both dressed in ill-fitting suits, with really weird short spiky hair full of wet-look gel. That cheap pink stuff you used to be able to buy from Superdrug. All I remember thinking was, *Quick! The girls are coming! Let's gel our hair!*

My overriding recollection of those first few years of having girls in my daily life at school is that it was hideous. I had absolutely no chill whatsoever. I've tried to forget as much as possible about those days but I can still make out vague outlines of memories. Embarrassingly asking girls out by *text* despite not knowing them very well, hovering around the ones that I fancied desperately trying to make them laugh in lessons and on one dreadful occasion, getting myself on the French trip to Lille even though I didn't even carry it on for upper sixth just so I could hang out with *REDACTED*. (I just can't do it to them or me.) We did hang out and had a nice time but she wasn't interested so I just spent the whole time trying to make her realise what she was missing out on while wandering around Christmas markets with the teacher. Harrowing.

I'm not entirely convinced that separating boys and girls in education is a great idea. The received wisdom is that boys can be very destructive, thereby affecting the grades of the girls and that's probably a good enough reason to keep us grotty lot away from them for as long as humanly possible – but the flip side for nervous dorks like me is that when the girls suddenly arrived, we didn't know what to do with ourselves. We went from spending five years laughing at each other's farts and doing wrestling moves at breaktime to suddenly having to share our school with what looked like grown women. Asking teenage boys to handle this well would be like asking adult humans to adapt to aliens in our midst. I was so inexperienced with girls that I didn't really understand the nuances that come with having a girlfriend or making friends that were girls. It just wasn't in my wheelhouse at all; I was profoundly unconfident in who I was back then. I just thought, mainly because of where society was at the time, that the only viable relationship with a girl was one where you had to be naked with them, and that's an incredibly narrow and potentially pretty damaging lens to look at women through.

The hair thing might seem trite but it's all connected. Back in sixth form, my insecurity about girls was mainly channelled into feeling like I had to do everything in my power to 'look good for the ladies', mainly in order to eventually end up playing with each other's genitals. This was a reductive way to see women for sure, born of lads' mags, the WWE Divas I mentioned earlier and a laddish popular culture that permeated the early noughties. Just as women's insecurities were exploited by companies wanting to sell them stuff, ours were used to tell us we weren't succeeding unless we were fighting women off. Those magazines in the early noughties were full of sexist language and images, the chocolate bar Yorkie was marketed using the infamous phrase 'IT'S NOT FOR GIRLS' and there were literally tits on Page Three of the

Sun newspaper *every day*. Tits in the paper! It wasn't a great time to be a teenager for either sex really. And no amount of hair gel could make me feel like I was attractive or suave.

The insecurities that my generation carried feel like they pale into insignificance compared to some of the women-hating, roid-taking, macho madness being spouted online now. This content is specifically aimed at teenage boys and young men, in ways that weren't available to those who came before, and it's frightening. A lot of the language in these male spaces is full of bravado, lacking a place for any vulnerability. This isn't in itself anything new. I grew up in a world where boys used insults and fighting as a way to form friendships too. I wasn't a particularly extreme example of this, though I absolutely would shape-shift into that role if I felt like it would help me fit in. I was mostly interested in traditionally softer, more creative spaces and activities, but I'd be lying if I said I hadn't joined in with some ridiculous laddy activity when the moment caught me. This kind of behaviour might always have been a way that boys bond, but it seems to have mushroomed and mutated, becoming far darker and more damaging for both the boys that take it in, and the women and girls around them.

The definition of 'masculinity' has always been very narrow (at least in this country), constraining men within arbitrary and made-up walls. It might be a stereotype to conjure up an image of lads as just wanting to achieve a six-pack, drink beer, watch footie (wheeeey lads), trip each other up and say someone's mum is fit, but it's not far off the truth. Of course there are millions of men who step outside these walls, but they can never fully escape the judgement of other men when they do. That's why it's so worrying to see young men listening to voices in the manosphere who are not only doubling down on ridiculous notions of masculinity, but adding new and awful lessons on what being a man is all about. We seemed to be moving away from this type of stuff in recent years but the language I hear increasingly on 'bro' podcasts seems to be harking back to that sad, pathetic time. Hustle culture, gym culture, grindset nonsense and Andrew fucking Tate being a misogynistic piece of shit very publicly, very loudly and very successfully is thoroughly depressing. Young boys are absorbing this stuff and it's sticking.

That should worry every single one of us, even those of us old enough to think we've escaped it. Masculinity might essentially be a made-up social construct, but the real-world impact is felt by everyone. It affects the way we react to women because most men have some level of ingrained sexism, even if we don't want to admit it. Take daily life: despite progress, gender roles are still so rigid. The chances are your mum probably did the washing, the cooking and the shopping, and your dad had the classically 'bigger' job that weighed heavy on life. This was certainly the case for me growing up. Despite my mum being an extraordinarily smart teacher, my dad's teaching career took off and therefore he earned more money, meaning that when he got promotions, we all had to up sticks and move. Of course, if my sister and I hadn't come along, who's to say that Mum wouldn't have been the one that became a headteacher? It's all hypothetical of course, but it's true to say that my own mum definitely had to find her way through a world that wasn't made for her.

As an adult, I've learnt that old-fashioned gender roles are important to be aware of in your own relationships. If you can't break the cycle entirely, you can at least redress some of the balance. Obviously Bella and I live in the same male-dominated world as everyone else, and my god do I have to be careful not to let my job dominate our lives. It's loud, it's invasive and it makes me tired and very grumpy sometimes. It's also out of the house whereas her job (author) is very much not, so invariably the majority of the domestic labour tends to fall at her door, which creates understandable tension. I grew up in a household where if Dad was stressed by his dominant job, we'd all feel it, and it fell to my mum to mollify him and make everything OK again. There's no way she would have wanted to do this but it's a role she would have felt forced to take on. I have to fight against this happening in my life and ensure that there's equal space for Bella, that she's not having to take on a maternal or 'fixer' role. I try to be very conscious not to make myself the larger person in the relationship. No one wants 'Greg James off the radio' at the dinner table every night. Not even me and I *am* him.

A lot of the way the world has been made has been by men, *for men*, and this only really became apparent to me when I made close friendships with girls. I've been fortunate to have been surrounded by brilliant role models, both men and women, who I could mess up in front of and learn from. It took me quite a few years to understand the complex power dynamics between men and women. Particularly young men and young women. Men tend to be stronger, a physical advantage that means they pose more of a threat than women – among numerous other benefits you get just by being born a boy. That's not to say that women aren't strong or capable, by the way, but the odds aren't usually in their favour. The anti-woke brigade will be worried that I've been radicalised into a snowflake by mad feminists or something, but then again, they're probably not reading this. They're probably listening to some podcast about tits and protein.

I wish I'd been told at a young age that being a straight white boy was going to mean I'd be first in the queue for lots of things, that people will tend to listen to me over anyone else (particularly women) and that I could get further ahead even when doing less work. If this had been calmly and clearly pointed out to me as a teenager, I hope I'd have taken it in and not become instantly defensive and angry just for being told I was lucky. Right now, a new version of masculinity is being fed to young boys, which tells them they're having their power stolen by women and minorities and that they need to fight back. Grifters like Tate have come along and created an army of radicalised morons fighting against an imaginary foe when all that those boys really need to know is that 'with great power (being a man) comes great responsibility'. Acknowledging you have an advantage and that things aren't always fair doesn't mean you lose anything, it just gives everyone the chance to fulfil their potential. You aren't being vilified or punished for being a man. Letting go of traditional ideas of masculinity doesn't just help women, it frees men too.

To turn back to your (or my) hair for a moment, ask what traditional masculinity has given you. It's probably given you an insecurity about your body, a constant worry about your hairline and a fear that women won't want to leap into bed with you. It's not serving anyone. So what should change? What will getting up at 4am, maximising your protein intake, blaming women and living by narrow rules invented by self-proclaimed macho gurus do for you? They're just giving you a list of unattainable objectives and providing you with a host of imaginary enemies to rail against, when you'll just end up railing against yourself and feeling sad and angry about the world.

I feel very lucky that my biggest male insecurity is just about my hair. I also feel lucky that I'm not a young boy being exposed to the rhetoric about how I need to train 15 times a week and be constantly on guard so that women don't try to take me down. On that subject, now would be a good time to practise what I preach and be a bit vulnerable and tell you some of the things I do as a man. I take finasteride every day to ensure I don't lose my hair as quickly as biology wants me to. I'm also currently doing Invisalign to make my teeth less wonky. I wear SPF every day, and do those strip things to make sure the pores on my nose are clean. I love having facials and pedicures and massages and sitting in the bath with bubbles and candles. I let the ladies at the nail place paint my toenails if they have time. I cry fairly often and always feel better after it. I tell all my male friends that I love them and put kisses on messages. I talk to them about their depression, their ADHD, their worries and insecurities. And other times we just sit and laugh at farts. I'm no more or less of a man for doing all this and the best advice is to ignore what society thinks about what you should look like or how you should act. Just be you (but don't be sexist).

What Would You Say to Your Younger Self?

I laugh so much when anyone gets asked this question. I get asked it a fair bit, and on the surface it sounds like it could solicit something profound. However, when it comes my way I have an overriding temptation to say, 'Well, the first thing I'd do is to question how the hell I've managed to meet little me and then once we'd established the mechanics of it, I'd spend a good amount of time calming down this presumably confused little child while trying to explain to him why a 40-year-old man is giving him advice.' More than anything, if we had managed to travel back in time, my first port of call wouldn't be to go and see eight-year-old me in 1990s Bromley. I just asked Bella what she'd do with this new time-travel superpower and she said, 'I'd go and see you in 1990s Bromley as a 41-year-old, find you in the park with your dad and say, "You're going to be my second husband and we're going to have a dog called Barney".' I'd have been excited about the dog bit but creeped out at the old lady that seemed to be part of the deal. I also think the answers you get to this question are often quite dull and trite. I should know, I've given a few of them and it's always been things like, 'Yeah, I'd tell him not to worry about girls. You'll get over your heartbreaks', 'You'll grow into your big pointy nose' (I did) and 'Your mum and dad aren't going to die before you're 20'.

I realise I'm wilfully misinterpreting the question a bit but one of the reasons I think it's pointless is because you *shouldn't* get too much advice when you're a kid. It's born out of a human instinct to 'make everything nice' and reassure someone you love. I often think this about my dog. If I could communicate verbally with him, I'd want to say, 'Don't worry, we're always going to come home again' or 'It's just the fucking postman, he's here every day, he's not about to plunder and pillage the house'. Although the house would be much quieter and we'd be a little less on edge, this would change his essence and that would be a shame. He would stop being a pure, chaotic, ridiculous dog and we don't want that. His dim-wittedness is what makes him brilliant. I don't want Barney to be rational because that's not what he is and it wouldn't be as fun. He is amazing at being a dog. It's like living with a cartoon; he's always in the moment and never dwelling on what happened yesterday or what's going to happen tomorrow. It doesn't matter to him because he's never thinking and nor do we want him to.

There's a temptation for humans to always want to meddle, and that's why the idea of visiting your younger self like some creepy old guardian angel is not only a pointless thought, but also unnecessary. All the things you do as a child, all the things you feel and experience, need to be colourful, unfiltered and, crucially, scary. This is how you learn about who you are and what you think and feel about things. We shouldn't tinker too much. You have to let things play out, not least because you don't have much choice in the matter.

Getting used to the discomfort of life is a huge part of being alive and we shouldn't shy away from that. I don't want to come across as a sadist but you only build resolve by going through some pain, grief or failure. I think a lot of us, particularly when we're young, have an unrealistic expectation that life is a simple straight line and that it's all going to work out well. Says who? That really isn't how it works and it's dangerous to think otherwise. All the things we've been taught lead us to think that if we follow these rules and learn these things then life will simply go well (cheers). It's like that for everyone. Some people are luckier than others, but you can't go through life without huge dollops of sadness landing at your door. I wasn't warned about how bleak and weird life can be or that we don't have much control over how our lives pan out. Kelly Clarkson famously taught us in 'Stronger' that what doesn't kill us makes us stronger, and as well as that song being an absolute banger, she's right. We need to build resilience to deal with the shit that gets thrown at us. You have to be proactive with it all and not be scared of it. Kelly also says, 'Because of you I learned to play on the safe side,' (also a banger) and this is a troubling place to operate from too. If anything, we should embrace the pain and the turmoil and then you're in a better position to take the wins when we can because you don't know when the next one's coming. Yes, there's great joy to be had in life, great happiness and great success, but you can't get the good without the bad. If intense elation comes along, you won't be able to truly enjoy it if you haven't also experienced acute sadness.

You can create an unhelpful narrative that everything and everyone is conspiring against you. I've been there: you have a bad day, everything and everyone is awful and you think someone's got it in for you. They haven't, of course. No one's got the time to set traps for you and if you start thinking that, you're not far off worrying that Bill Gates is spying on you through vaccines or whatever those fucking cranks think. Bill Gates is too busy curing polio and designing a new update for Excel or whatever he does now to worry about what Martin in Dartford's doing in his bedroom. It's perhaps more comforting to think that there's a plan for you and that there is someone controlling your destiny but there really isn't. I've tried really hard over the last few years to get into the habit of shrugging things off. There's great power in giving less energy to the shit that doesn't go right.

Perhaps I do have some good advice not just for my younger self, but for anyone: don't be alarmed when things go tits up. That's how it's supposed to be and the world isn't against you. Especially you, Martin. Also, my advice to you is pull your trousers up and go get some fresh air.

That being said, if anyone asks me the question in the future (and they will), these are now the only answers I will give:

1.   Go and see a doctor. Hearing an old version of you talking about the future isn't a good sign.
2.   You won't be able to work out how to do your hair properly until you're 35 and then you'll become really obsessed with it to the point it's a banned talking point in the house.
3.   You'll never be happy with a single photograph of yourself. And nor should you be. Stay humble and don't be a monster.
4.   The wind will become your nemesis.
5.   So will Heart 106.2.

6. Lots of the people you liked on TV in the 1990s will reveal themselves to be quite odd.

7. Everyone will laugh at how much we panicked about the Millenium Bug.

8. No man looks comfortable holding a tote bag.

9. You know those very niche podcasts you like? Well, they will become mainstream, which is great news; however, it also means that the most annoying people in the world will discover that doing one will make them a quick buck – but don't worry, they'll get bored and do something else after a couple of years.

10. You'll be tempted to stare moronically at your phone for hours on end and learn nothing.

11. When you hit 30, it is unavoidable that worrying about where to park becomes a thing.

12. You don't need to wash your clothes as often as you think you do.

13. You're going to be scared of birds flapping around your head and your wife will think it's hilarious (it's not).

14. You'll become best friends with a dog.

15. You won't mind picking up his disgusting shits and you'll take pride in ones that are healthy because it means he's being looked after well.

16. You will really really love wine.

17. It's OK to stop being friends with people. That's part of life. In fact, you'll keep making new ones as you get older.

18. Oh, that one was a bit earnest ... how about ... you'll regret not sticking with piano lessons.

19. Still a bit serious … urm … You'll think about Lenin more than you want to. We did a school trip to Russia in 2001 and we saw his embalmed yellow body lying in state and it was one of the funniest things I've ever seen. It pops into my head too much. OK, that was less serious, but quite odd. Do a funny one.
20. You'll write a critically acclaimed *Sunday Times* bestseller. There. Nailed it.

Cheap laughs aside, I sit here today pretty near the end of writing my first solo book feeling like a bigger, smarter version of the little boy that appeared at the start with his nan in Weymouth waiting for the Chuckle Brothers. Would the young me like the current me?

Even though we're not asking what you'd say to your younger self, I think the younger me would like what's happened to the older him. He'd see that he was trying to be the best friend I can be to the people I love the most in the world, that I do all I can to make sure I'm wholeheartedly throwing everything I have into this amazing marriage I have with Bella and making sure I'm supporting her as much as I can. He'd also love how close I still am to his parents – how often I go and watch sport with Dad and how I still like helping Mum out in the garden, and he'd be so impressed that he gets to boss his big scary sister around like she used to do to him. But also that he can now buy *her* nice dinners like she used to do for me when I was a lowly student. He'd be so excited to know that I can buy myself an electric train set if I want to, that I managed to get a job talking about cricket which means I get to go to basically any game and that I'm friends with Jimmy Anderson. He'd find it hard to get his head around the fact that I've driven some of the best cars in the world. And of course, young Greg would be amazed that old Greg managed to do a job that he dreamt of doing, he'd be obsessed with Barney and he'd be floored that I have Paul Chuckle's phone number and that I was about to go and meet him. What?! I'm going to meet him? Where else did you think the book was going? It's not just thrown together, you know ...

Me,
to
Him

I'm walking with purpose across the concourse of St Pancras station after the *Breakfast Show*. I escaped a little earlier than usual because I'm on a mission. A mission I'm incredibly excited about. The train is at 11.35. I look at my phone. It's 11.22. I've got plenty of time to get a coffee and a pain au chocolat from Paul (the bakery) and even enough time to send a selfie to Bella in front of the PAUL sign, as I always do because it's the name of her ex-husband and it's never not funny. The joke started quite early on in our relationship when we were going away somewhere and she declared she was 'going to Paul'. 'Paul LEFT YOU,' I declared. It was risky but it paid off. She immediately erupted into laughter and it's been a running 'bit' ever since. Her sister even gets in on the act. There is no mercy, but that's love.

It's early December and as I make my way past the twinkly window displays towards platform 2, I pass all the smug wankers in fake fur coats holding Longchamp bags heading off to Paris for a bout of Christmas shopping and a saunter down the Champs-Élysées. I would usually feel incredibly jealous of them but I'm off to do something much better. Something unique. I'm off to meet Paul Chuckle. It will be the first time I've seen him face-to-face since that perfect day in 1996.

The last time I saw this man was 30 years ago when he handed me that signed photo of him and his brother which said, 'All the best for the future'. I looked out of the train window (pensively of course, while listening to Sam Fender) and it hit me that this is quite a significant moment. I feel weirdly emotional about it. I think of Weymouth and of my nan, I think of those summer holidays where I didn't need to achieve anything other than watch cartoons and eat toasted cheese sandwiches. I think of the road trips down there, the beach, the amusement arcades, of my youthful parents paying for yet another go on the bumper boats and of my open-eyed excitement and naivety at the world. I wonder how much of that boy is still me. How much have I changed? In 1996, I didn't really know of any of the horrors of life. I was blissfully unaware of the evils that were lurking. Things that as a grown-up you just have to get used to: war, fascists, heartbreak, the *Diary Of A CEO* podcast. Despite knowing more about the sad offerings life presents us with, I still get excited by things in the same way I did back then. You perhaps have to look a little harder, squint past the sadness, but you can still find them. Thinking about my childhood has made me fall into a nostalgia vortex. I luxuriated in it for a second too long and inevitably got sad about all my favourite people dying so I've broken myself out of it by looking at my phone for a cheap distraction.

I'm back now and wondering whether I really miss the old days or whether it's a trick of memory. I do a bit, I've decided. But I don't wish away my life now. I've learnt to enjoy the passing of time, the friendships that come along and fade away, the relationships that broke my heart but helped me make sense of who I was and who I am. And like I say, I don't think I've lost that wide-eyed excitement I had as a kid. I mean, I'm on a train to meet one of the fucking Chuckle Brothers, having centred my debut non-fiction book around them, so I think that's quite clear.

Paul Chuckle seemed to like ten-year-old me, but will he like 38-year-old me? Let's find out. The train is about to pull into the station; it's a bright, chilly day in the East Midlands which is a relief after yet another weekend of storms that caused widespread floods. I'm gliding past large bodies of water which are hiding the farm-land beneath. The sun glistens off the surface and although things aren't as they're supposed to be, the fields seem to be enjoying their new role as great lakes.

I'm also enjoying my new role as a non-fiction author as I bundle myself and my rucksack full of notes into a cab and head for Paul's rented apartment just on the edge of Nottingham. The reason he's there is because he's playing the role of the foppish Starkey in the Theatre Royal's *Peter Pan*(tomime) alongside Denise Welch and Gok Wan. Good line-up, to be fair. As I walk up to the communal doors, I call Paul on WhatsApp. Even having his phone number feels mad to me. The whole thing's mad. It's yet another great lesson in following your instincts, saying yes to the funny thing and prior-itising having a nice time. I think (and hope) that Paul shares these values. I'm pretty sure he does because otherwise he wouldn't have agreed to chat to me for a book about that central message.

You can see the lift from the front door of the apartment block and as the door slides open, one of the most recognisable faces in the country appears, beaming, bespectacled as he gives me a big showbiz wave. 'Great to finally meet you,' we both say in harmony. I really meant it, too. It really *was* great to meet him. A childhood hero, a person who made me realise silly was funny, funny was silly and that silly was good. A good way to approach life. Maybe it's the best way, no, the *only* way to get through it. I'm sure we'll get into that.

For now though, I find myself crammed into a lift with a Chuckle Brother. His face in real life is somehow even kinder and friendlier than on the TV. I immediately feel comfortable with him; he has a quiet, calm charisma that puts me at ease and there isn't even a hint of not wanting to bother with all this. And believe me, I've interviewed enough celebrities to know when they can't be arsed. We get off on the third floor and walk down the corridors to get to his door. His wife of nearly 40 years, Sue, is waiting at the door and I'm ushered in. 'I'm staying here until the 12th of January. It's a long run. Knackering. Fun though!' *Christ*, I think. *That IS a long run.* Two shows a day, 12 shows a week. The man's 77! 'You must love it!' I say, somewhat naively. 'I do! Money's good, too,' he replies, cheekily. I find out that there's been drama before the run's properly started. Apparently Denise Welch is unwell and has to pull out of the entire run, and they've drafted in Richard Winsor from *Casualty* as cover. As well as that, Gok Wan's been ill so the director had to go on and do his part while reading the lines from the script. Paul says the audience sympathised massively and the show was 'great'. I bet it was, as well. 'The show must go on!' Paul says, 'you've got to give 100 per cent every time you go out there. Wherever you are.' This, I begin to realise, is one of the main secrets to his success. There he was, a man who's been in show business since 1963, the eldest member of the cast, on a cold night in Nottingham in December, holding it all together on opening night one. 'I was the only name left on the bill!'

As we begin to talk, I realise that their long and arduous road to national treasure status is the thing that gave them not only their resilience but also an astonishing work ethic. Fame came relatively late to Paul and Barry after years of hard graft in various comedy venues, working men's clubs, summer seasons around the UK, endless pantomimes, guest spots on TV and then eventually their big break with *ChuckleVision* in 1987. I realise that the man I met in 1996 in Weymouth with my nan would have been in his late forties. He was married and had kids by then but still had so much energy, so much life and so much fun. In my head they were 20, but in reality they would have been older than my parents at the time. Again, age has nothing to do with it. It's all about youthfulness. You can't help getting older, but you can help getting *old*.

As I'm about to sit down to start the interview, I realise I have to shuffle one of the chairs so I'm facing Paul and I resist the temptation to drop a 'To Me! To You!' Who will be the first to do it? Sue offers me coffee and a delicious bacon sandwich and we get chatting. I start off by asking him about the title of this book you have in your hands. Did he like doing those meet and greets with smelly little twerps like me? 'It was always great. Meeting your fans one-to-one is always a lovely feeling. I love that feeling of love and warmth from a crowd. It makes you feel proud of what you've made,' he replies, smiling. I ask him if he often wrote 'All the best for the future' to ten-year-olds. 'No!' He laughs. 'You must have said something for me to reply with that. Maybe you said you were going to do this when you grew up or something?'

I *was* completely obsessed with theatre and special effects and stunts and lighting and smoke machines and all that nonsense as a little boy (and still very much am) so I tell Paul that this is entirely plausible. Either way, it was a funny thing to write to a kid. And it stuck with me.

He speaks so fondly of those summer seasons at Weymouth Pavilion, 'Oh, I loved it,' he says. 'We were there Monday, Tuesday, Wednesday and then we went and did other things but for those three days we stayed in Weymouth. Fabulous place. I remember they gave us a watercolour painting of the harbour. It's on the wall at home.' I start beaming. Is he just telling me what I want to hear? Does he realise he has my childhood memories in the palm of his hand or is he just a genuinely good man? I'm sure it's the latter. Paul's memory is in glorious technicolour and the recollections are accessed so quickly and succinctly but with no lack of emotion. It's a real pleasure to be listening to him.

I wonder what Paul's dreams were when he was a kid and he very quickly replies, 'I wanted to be a footballer'. This is the first time I detect sadness from Chuckle the Younger. 'I was devastated when I got injured.' His leg didn't ever heal properly and he tells me that he just couldn't get up to speed again afterwards. 'We had a fabulous football team,' he continues, 'for three seasons in the senior school, we were unbeaten. And when we left school at fifteen, eight of my mates turned professional. I would have been the ninth if it wasn't for the injury. My mate Phil went on to play for Sheffield United.' 'You wouldn't have exchanged that for the career you went on to have, would you?!' I ask. 'Well, I could have had both because I was 39 when Chuckle Brothers started!'

I laugh because he knows he's being dramatic. I point out that without the 20-odd years of learning his trade and perfecting his craft in the working men's clubs and holiday parks, he and Barry wouldn't have been in a position to become the Chuckle Brothers. He of course also knows this but I find it interesting that even when people ended up doing the job they *should* be doing, there's always another dream that came before it. It's beautifully childlike to still believe deep down that you could have been a footballer. 'I could have done second division,' he adds. I tell him that I can relate to this as I was once convinced that I should open the batting for England. To my surprise he tells me that he opened the batting for his school team but shyness and lack of confidence put paid to any cricketing dreams. 'This was exactly my problem!' I declare. We're kindred spirits.

I ask Paul about growing up in the public eye and how he managed to balance not only the knockbacks of life but also the knockbacks of a career in entertainment. 'If anything went wrong on stage, we'd just have fun because we had each other.' On the trappings of showbiz, he points out that they already had a solid base from years of working the clubs, so when they got famous, they avoided drink and drugs because it would have been mad to throw it all away after such hard graft. Paul talks beautifully about being humble and generous to fellow performers and the people you work with: 'You have to always be nice to people on your way up because they'll be nice to you on the way down. If you're nasty and big-headed and what have you, as soon as you're done nobody wants to know you. Like Cannon and Ball – they were awful people.' I laugh at this because firstly I didn't know there was a rivalry but secondly, I hadn't considered that the Chuckle Brothers were capable of this level of showbiz bitching. It's fantastic and makes me like Paul even more. I remember the thing I keep banging on about in this book about nobody being just one thing. I'm sure a few of you are surprised I dislike lots of things, but personally I love it when someone calls a cunt a cunt.

I point out that a lot of life happens while you're out there performing and the trick is to never really let on to the audience that your mind is elsewhere. Life delivers its own custard pies to the face while you're doing them on stage. It's quite hard to hide that sadness when your brother is your sidekick and he dies. Everyone notices. And everyone points it out. 'The first thing we did [when Barry died] was go on a three-week holiday to China,' Paul says, 'I wanted to go somewhere where people weren't coming up to me saying that they're sorry to hear about Barry and in China, not one person knew who I was.' After excitedly telling me about Shanghai and their adventures there, we're back in the UK again and he recollects walking through the airport where people were still coming up to him wanting to speak about Barry. 'I felt a bit rude at times, because you didn't want to get into a conversation as you'd feel the tears coming.' I realise suddenly that we do absolutely insane jobs. No matter what happens to you, everyone that meets you expects the person they see on stage, watch on TV or hear on the radio. You're always on. Like the sun or *The Chase* with Bradley Walsh. And even if you're behind a cloud, trapped in the biggest, saddest storm, you've still got to shine. Yes, it would have been tricky for Paul, but actually, what a privilege. It's truly wonderful that people care that much to want to speak to you, to share a memory or their condolences. In any job, you've still got to put on a show of sorts. It's interesting to me that even in his deepest despair at his brother – a part of him – dying, he's still worried about coming across as rude to people in the street. The audience comes first, though. And also, crucially, this is Paul's job. This is his income. He loves to work, sure, but like most people, he also has to.

Four months after Barry's death, he was back on stage in Craig Revel Horwood's pantomime, *Cinderella*. 'Since I was fifteen, I always had Barry with me doing the funny lines and me giving him the feed and we'd always come on either side of the stage, meet in the middle, walk down to the front and do a double take as if we were surprised people were there ...' I'm suddenly ten years old again. I remember this 'bit' vividly. It's a great bit. Paul continues, 'I had to do it on my own that first night without Barry and to this day I swear I saw Barry on the other side of the stage before the music started, giving me a thumbs up. As I walked out on stage, the place erupted, it was huge. He'd only died four months before and I hoped it wasn't sympathy but they laughed at everything I did. They were brilliant and it's been the same since. All these years later.'

I pause for a moment to take in what's just been said. One of the saddest but most poignant things I've ever heard. Deeply tragic but beautifully uplifting. It's easy to trivialise silly things like the Chuckle Brothers but if that's not a perfect example of togetherness and community then I don't know what is. I felt it that day back in 1996. They wanted me to be part of their gang. That's what they wanted for everyone who watched them.

They were there for us after school every day, messing around to make us laugh, so of course that audience was there when he needed them. When Paul walked out on his own in that first show without Barry, people wanted to show up for him when he needed it. I feel incredibly fortunate to be listening to him tell me all this and I'm also relieved that he is as together and normal as I'd hoped. It's brilliant and reassuring, as a fan, to realise that the funny, silly, charismatic performer you've grown up watching also has a real life. He has a sturdy base from which to operate. A loving family, hobbies and interests away from work, a love of travel – he's waxing lyrical about a mega cruise they went on, a surprise trip to Brooklyn they recently took, their annual holiday to Benidorm at Easter, a pilgrimage to one of their villas in Greece … No wonder he has to keep working! He lives a nice life! And it makes me incredibly happy.

We've been chatting for about 90 minutes and although I could do another 90, I think it's best to leave him in peace. It's his last day off before the run properly gets going, after all. As we rattle down to the ground floor, Sue mentions something innocuous to Paul that I semi-hear but notice that it included the phrasing '… to me' at the end of the sentence. Paul, as quick as a flash, instinctively says '… to you!' and I burst out laughing. He did it! It was ridiculous. He's still very much got it. That childlike silliness, the perfect comedy timing, the ability to make someone crack up by doing the daftest thing, pulling a funny face or simply saying the words 'to you'. They both give me a big hug at the door as I wait for the cab back to the station. Sue presents me with a copy of Paul and Barry's 2014 book, which celebrated 50 years of them performing together, which is a lovely gesture. In fact, such is their warmth that I sort of feel like their long-lost son, being waved off after a long-overdue visit.

I'm sitting on the train again. Off I go back to my life, as he goes back to his. I open the book that Sue handed me. It's signed! 'To Gregory, All the best in the future,' is written in Paul's handwriting. Perfect. Made even better by the fact that he's got it slightly wrong. But I ponder it for a second. What does 'all the best for the future' mean to me now? What did it mean to me then? Is it just a funny anecdote that I've periodically told throughout my life and thought strong enough to make the title of my book? A bit, yes. But there's something quite comforting about it that has only really become apparent through writing this book and also meeting the man who wrote it on a photograph 30 years ago. All the things you've ever done, seen or been through make up not just the present, but also the future. The idea of 'the future' is too vast to think of as a goal or a destination. It's also the wrong way to approach it. The future is everything you do from this moment.

Life is made up of the tiny bits. Minute by minute. A decision here, a decision there. Some right, some wrong, some mundane, some unimportant, some huge, some vital. But really, there is no point worrying about the macro. Focus on the micro. I could never have imagined how my life has currently ended up and neither could Paul imagine his. He just did what he thought was right in the moment and his future happened regardless. That's how all of our futures end up. They just happen, and all you can do is what you think is right day by day. Don't dismiss the small, boring moments. The day spent watching your favourite show and eating crisps, a rambling phone call with a mate, a solo trip to the seaside, a three-hour bath. They're all part of the whole. The only way you can get to the future is by experiencing all that life throws at you. All you have to do is try to make it through in one piece, full of things you've learnt, lost, regretted, enjoyed, hated, laughed at and cried at, but crucially, experienced and *survived*. As that ten-year-old boy, I had no idea about all the things that were in my future and neither did Paul. But he knew the future would come and with it a whole avalanche of different emotions and experiences. Some great, some tragic. But when you're doing the audit of your life one day nearer the end, if you're lucky, you'll be able to look back and see there's been a net gain.

On the train, I flick to the foreword, which was written by the legendary comic Ken Dodd. 'The Chuckle Brothers are what real entertainment is all about,' he says. 'They sing, they dance, they act and they are very, very funny … That is real showbusiness.' They also prioritised fun whenever they got the chance. In between the serious bits of life was a lot of joy. You can always find the fun. Life is absurd and sometimes it deserves to be laughed at. That's a great lesson to all of us.

Your Nemeses

1 ....

2 ....

3 ....

4 ....

5 ....

6 ....

7 ....

8 ....

9 ....

10 ....

Unpopular Opinions

The things the world says you should like but you don't ...

- ....

....

- ....

....

- ....

....

- ....

....

- ....

....

- ....

....

Your Perfect Waste Day

Morning ....

....

Mid-morning ....

....

Midday ....

....

Mid-afternoon ....

....

Evening ....

....

Night ....

....

A Place to List Your Worries
(Big and Small)

- ....

  ....

- ....

  ....

- ....

  ....

- ....

  ....

- ....

  ....

- ....

  ....

Acknowledgements

Writing a book is often seen as a solo effort and while the physical act of figuring out what you want to say and typing out the words (not to mention having multiple existential crises) is on you as the author, it takes a real team to bring the whole thing together. It's been incredibly joyful and fulfilling to work with and learn from a group of people at the top of their industry. I am very, very lucky.

Firstly – and mainly – this book would not have happened without the support, guidance, friendship, patience, skill, humour and intelligence of my editor, Charlotte Hardman. It's been a real pleasure to form a double act with you over the last couple of years. Perhaps we could be the new Chuckle Brothers one day. I'll be forever in your debt. And also thank you for helping pay off some of my debt with the advance. To everyone else at Penguin for their support, I'm forever proud to be one of your authors. Very proud little penguin over here. The team at Ebury have made this book better in a thousand different ways. Thank you to Loulou Clark, Shelise Robertson, Shasmin Mozomil, Lucy Brown, Patsy O'Neill, Jasmin Kaur, Jessica Anderson, Aslan Byrne (greatest name in the game), Rachel Myers, Ben Green, Beth Stuart, Tracy Orchard, Jade Perez, Percie Bridgewater, Alfie Thompson and Hannah Cawse. I hope you feel proud of what we've all made. If it's received with even a tenth of the love, kindness and enthusiasm that it was made with, I'll be happy.

Elsewhere, I'd like to thank my dazzling wife, Bella, for being a constant cheerleader and sounding board for all the ideas I threw into this (thank you for vetoing the shit ones). Felix White, who inspires me constantly with what he creates. Fe, that chat at the cricket helped me bring the whole book together, thank you. Chris Sawyer, thank you not only for the nonsense we're about to undertake in the next few weeks to sell the damn thing, but for giving me the confidence to express myself and for making me funnier and better. Thank you Mattchin for being so keen to read it before it was ready and for your unexpectedly detailed notes, which genuinely helped. Thank you Dad for also being one of the first to read it and for returning it like a piece of coursework with suggestions. The main one being 'you say "actually" too much'. And *actually* he was right. Parents always are. The number of actuallys have been dramatically reduced in this final draft. A very special thank you to Paul Elliot (Chuckle) and his wonderful wife, Sue, for being willing and excited to be involved from the very start. What a very brilliant, generous man. A very special thank you to Merope Mills and Paul Laity, as well as Martha's wonderful little sister, Lottie. Thank you to all of you for your friendship and also for letting me write about your amazing daughter.

Thank you also to my literary agent, Steph Thwaites. We started cooking up the loose idea for this book a long time ago and I'm so grateful you barged your way into my life. I hope you like it! You've helped me achieve things I didn't think possible. You're great. Thank you also to everybody else at Curtis Brown, and in particular to Meryl Hoffman. Your patience and support while I went mad and cancelled every other bit of work to prioritise this bloody book will never be forgotten. Thank you to my wonderful *Breakfast Show* team, along with Lorna, Aled and Pete, who have all been across what I've written in here and let me get away with pretty much all of it so yeah lets see how that all goes shall we? Everyone at Radio 1 makes coming into work and creating fun things for our listeners the greatest pleasure. I love working there and I love you all very much. We trade in joy and I feel so lucky to be surrounded by such brilliant, silly, chaotic brains.

And, finally, to my very close friends and family. My nearest and dearest. I love you all so much. You always encourage me to live the way I've spent 300 pages telling everyone else how to. Let's keep that up, please.